RANSOM KHANYE

Garlic

Nature's Miracle Clove

Cover design by Ransom Khanye
All copyrights reserved.

No portion of this book may be reproduced in any form without written permission from the author.

ISBN:9798883027481

Also available on Amazon, about natural remedies, and by the same author:

1. **The Magic Oil: Unleashing the Power of Nature's Remedy - Castor Oil**
2. **The Magic Oil 2: More Castor Oil Miracles**
3. **Amazing Natural Remedies: Nature's Medicine Cabinet**
4. **101 Castor Oil Recipes for Health and Beauty: The Complete Guide to Castor Oil Remedies**
5. **The Root of Health: Ginseng**
6. **The Red Hot Remedy: The Ultimate Guide to Cayenne Pepper Benefits**

[Note: This book does not make claims to diagnose, treat, or cure any specific diseases or medical conditions. It is intended for informational purposes only and should not replace professional medical advice or treatment.]

Garlic

FOREWORD

Welcome, dear reader, to the captivating world of "Garlic: Nature's Miracle Clove". As you hold this book in your hands, you're embarking on a journey into the extraordinary realm of one of nature's most remarkable gifts: garlic.

In this meticulously crafted volume, I invite you to explore the rich tapestry of garlic's history, its myriad of health benefits, and its versatile culinary applications. From ancient civilizations to modern scientific research, garlic has stood the test of time as a symbol of vitality, wellness, and culinary delight.

As you delve into this book, you'll uncover the ancient wisdom surrounding garlic's use, from folklore and mythology to its esteemed place in traditional medicine systems. You'll gain insights into the science behind garlic's healing powers, unlocking the secrets of its potent compounds and their effects on the human body.

But this book is more than just a compendium of facts and figures—it's a celebration of garlic in all its forms. You'll journey through the world of garlic cultivation, explore its diverse varieties and flavors, and discover tantalizing recipes from kitchens around the globe.

Whether you're seeking to boost your immune system, improve your heart health, or simply elevate your culinary creations, "Garlic: Nature's Miracle Clove" is your indispensable guide. Through its pages, you'll learn how to harness the power of garlic to enhance every aspect of your life, from wellness to gastronomy. So let this book be your companion on a voyage of discovery, as you unlock the secrets of this humble yet extraordinary herb.

With warmest regards,
Ransom Khanye

Garlic

5

Contents

Chapter 1: The Ancient Wisdom: Garlic through the Ages

In the history of humanity, very few ingredients have woven themselves into the fabric of civilization quite like garlic. From the sun-baked lands of ancient Egypt to the bustling markets of medieval Europe, garlic has been revered not only for its culinary prowess but also for its myriad of medicinal and mystical properties.

Under the shadows of the majestic pyramids, garlic emerged as a staple of ancient Egyptian culture, revered for both its flavor and its perceived protective powers. Believed to bestow strength and ward off evil spirits, garlic adorned the tombs of pharaohs and accompanied the departed on their journey to the so called "afterlife".

Across the shimmering waters of the Mediterranean, the Greeks and Romans embraced garlic with equal fervor. Renowned for its ability to invigorate the body and sharpen the mind, garlic found its place in the annals of ancient medicine, prescribed by healers and philosophers alike.

As the Roman legions marched across Europe, they carried with them not only swords and shields but also bulbs of garlic, prized for their ability to fortify soldiers against disease and infection. In the bustling markets of Rome, garlic adorned the stalls of merchants, its pungent aroma mingling with the scent of spices and exotic wares.

In the hallowed halls of medieval monasteries, garlic took on new significance as monks cultivated its aromatic bulbs in cloistered gardens. Revered for its ability to cleanse both body and soul, garlic became a staple of monastic cuisine and herbal remedies, its pungent aroma wafting through the corridors of medieval abbeys.

As Europe emerged from the shadows of the Middle Ages, garlic found itself at the center of a culinary renaissance, celebrated by chefs and gourmands alike. From the sumptuous feasts of Renaissance Italy to the rustic taverns of medieval England, garlic infused the dishes of kings and commoners alike, its bold flavor transforming humble meals into epicurean delights.

Yet, beyond its culinary and medicinal prowess, garlic has always held a deeper significance for humanity—a symbol of strength, resilience, and protection against the vagaries of fate. From the sands of ancient Egypt to the cobblestone streets of medieval Europe, garlic has endured as a testament to the enduring power of nature's bounty.

In the chapters that follow, we will delve deeper into the mysteries of garlic, exploring its ancient wisdom and uncovering the secrets of its timeless allure. Through the lens of history, we will sojourn across continents and centuries, tracing the path of garlic from a humble herb to a revered icon.

Sources:
- Davidson, Alan. The Oxford Companion to Food. Oxford University Press, 2014.
- Purcell, William M. "Garlic: A Survey of Its Historic and Medicinal Uses." HerbalGram, no. 44, 1998, pp. 33–48.
- Simon, Reeva S., et al. The Jews of Medieval Western Christendom, 1000-1500. Cambridge University Press, 1996.

Chapter 2: Unveiling Garlic's Healing Powers

In the quiet corners of ancient apothecaries and the bustling laboratories of modern science, garlic has long been celebrated as nature's elixir—a potent panacea endowed with a myriad of healing powers. From the fields of ancient Egypt to the cutting-edge clinics of today, garlic has earned its place as a cornerstone of natural medicine, revered for its ability to soothe, strengthen, and heal.

At the heart of garlic's healing prowess lie its remarkable bioactive compounds—powerful phytochemicals that imbue this humble herb with its distinctive flavor and aroma. Chief among these compounds is **allicin**, a sulfur-containing compound that has been the focus of much scientific inquiry. Allicin is released when garlic cloves are crushed or chopped, unleashing a cascade of biochemical reactions that give garlic its characteristic pungency and therapeutic potency.

But allicin is just the beginning. Garlic boasts a veritable treasure trove of bioactive compounds, including **diallyl sulfide**, **diallyl disulfide**, and **ajoene**, each with its own unique set of health-promoting properties. Together, these compounds work in harmony to combat inflammation, boost the immune system, and protect against a host of ailments.

Scientific studies have provided compelling evidence of garlic's medicinal benefits, validating the wisdom of ancient healers and herbalists. Research has shown that garlic possesses potent antimicrobial properties, capable of inhibiting the growth of bacteria, viruses, and fungi. In clinical trials, garlic has been found to be effective against a wide range of pathogens, including antibiotic-resistant strains—a testament to its enduring relevance in the fight against infectious disease.

But garlic's healing powers extend far beyond its antimicrobial properties. Studies have shown that garlic can help lower cholesterol levels, reduce blood pressure, and improve cardiovascular health. Its anti-inflammatory effects make it a valuable ally in the fight against chronic diseases such as arthritis and diabetes. And emerging research suggests that garlic may even play a role in cancer prevention, with studies pointing to its ability to inhibit tumor growth and protect against DNA damage.

Yet perhaps the most remarkable aspect of garlic's healing powers is its versatility. Whether consumed raw, cooked, or in supplement form, garlic offers a potent arsenal of natural remedies for a wide range of ailments. From colds and flu to chronic conditions like asthma and arthritis, garlic stands ready to offer relief—a testament to the enduring wisdom of nature's pharmacy.

In the chapters that follow, we will delve deeper into the remarkable healing powers of garlic, exploring its diverse array of health benefits and practical applications. Through the lens of science and tradition, we will unlock the secrets of this extraordinary herb, revealing the timeless wisdom of garlic as nature's most potent healer.

Sources:
- Bayan, Leyla, et al. "Garlic: A review of potential therapeutic effects." Avicenna Journal of Phytomedicine, vol. 4, no. 1, 2014, pp. 1–14.
- Rahman, Khalid, and Fazal-ur-Rehman Bhatti. "Garlic (Allium sativum): a review of its adverse effects on health." Journal of Toxicology and Environmental Health Sciences, vol. 4, no. 1, 2012, pp. 1–6.
- Reinhart, Karen M., and Christine M. Coleman. "Garlic: Source of the Ultimate Anti-cancer Compound - A Review." Current Drug Metabolism, vol. 9, no. 4, 2008, pp. 393–397.

Chapter 3: Garlic in Folklore and Mythology

In human culture, garlic occupies a hallowed place, its pungent aroma and potent flavor woven into the very fabric of folklore and mythology. Across continents and centuries, garlic has been revered not only for its culinary and medicinal properties but also for its mystical and symbolic significance—a humble herb elevated to the status of a sacred talisman.

Journey with me now as we delve into the captivating realm of garlic in folklore and mythology, where tales of magic, mystery, and the supernatural intertwine with the everyday lives of ordinary people.

Exploration of Garlic's Mythological and Cultural Significance
Garlic's journey through the annals of myth and legend begins in the ancient civilizations of the Mediterranean, where it was revered as a symbol of strength, protection, and vitality. In ancient Egypt, garlic adorned the tombs of pharaohs, believed to ward off evil spirits and ensure safe passage to the afterlife. In Greece and Rome, garlic was consecrated to the gods, its potent aroma believed to bestow courage and invigorate the body.

Legends and Stories Featuring Garlic from Different Cultures
From the sun-drenched shores of the Mediterranean to the misty mountains of Asia, garlic has left an indelible mark on the collective imagination of humanity. In China, garlic is celebrated as a symbol of prosperity and good fortune, its bulbs hung above doorways to ward

off malevolent spirits. In Eastern Europe, garlic is said to possess the power to repel vampires and other supernatural creatures, its pungent aroma serving as a potent deterrent against the forces of darkness.

Superstitions and Beliefs Associated with Garlic
Throughout history, garlic has been imbued with a myriad of superstitions and beliefs, ranging from the protective to the prophylactic. In medieval Europe, garlic was worn as an amulet to ward off disease and protect against malevolent spirits. In ancient Greece, garlic was believed to confer strength and courage upon warriors, who consumed it before battle to ensure victory.

Garlic's Portrayal in Literature, Art, and Folklore
From the pages of ancient texts to the canvases of master painters, garlic has been immortalized in literature, art, and folklore. In the works of Shakespeare, garlic is mentioned as a potent remedy for ailing spirits, its aroma believed to dispel melancholy and restore vitality. In the paintings of Renaissance masters, garlic appears as a symbol of abundance and prosperity, its golden bulbs evoking the bounty of the earth.

As we traverse through the realm of garlic in folklore and mythology, let us pause to savor the richness of its lore and the depth of its symbolism. For in the humble bulb of garlic, we find not only sustenance for the body but nourishment too — a reminder of the enduring power of myth and legend to illuminate the human experience.

Sources:
- Dundes, Alan. "Garlic as a Protective Charm." The Journal of American Folklore, vol. 83, no. 328, 1970, pp. 48–50.
- Roud, Steve. The Penguin Guide to the Superstitions of Britain and Ireland. Penguin Books, 2003.
- Sanecki, Kay, and Kay Sanecki. Garlic: The Mighty Bulb. Houghton Mifflin Harcourt, 1997.

Chapter 4: The Science Behind Garlic's Health Benefits

In the pursuit of understanding garlic's remarkable healing powers, we take a trip into the realm of science—a realm where molecules and mechanisms converge to unravel the mysteries of this humble herb's therapeutic potential. Join me as we delve into the intricate world of garlic's chemical composition and the fascinating mechanisms that underpin its myriad health benefits.

Detailed Explanation of Garlic's Chemical Composition
At the heart of garlic's medicinal prowess lies its complex chemical composition, a symphony of organic compounds that imbue this unassuming herb with its distinctive flavor and aroma. From allicin to diallyl sulfides, garlic boasts a rich array of sulfur-containing compounds, each contributing to its therapeutic potency.

Breakdown of Allicin and Other Sulfur Compounds in Garlic
Chief among garlic's bioactive constituents is allicin, a sulfur-containing compound that is formed when garlic cloves are crushed or chopped. Allicin is responsible for garlic's characteristic pungency and is believed to be a key player in many of its health-promoting effects. In addition to allicin, garlic also contains a variety of other sulfur compounds, including **diallyl sulfides** and **ajoene**, each with its own unique set of properties.

Mechanisms of Action Behind Garlic's Therapeutic Effects

The therapeutic effects of garlic are mediated by a multitude of mechanisms, acting on everything from the cardiovascular system to the immune response. Allicin, for example, has been shown to exhibit potent antimicrobial properties, inhibiting the growth of bacteria, viruses, and fungi. Other sulfur compounds in garlic have been found to exert anti-inflammatory, antioxidant, and anticancer effects, making garlic a true powerhouse of natural medicine.

Overview of Scientific Research Supporting Garlic's Health Benefits

Decades of scientific research have provided compelling evidence of garlic's myriad health benefits, validating the wisdom of traditional healers and herbalists. Clinical studies have demonstrated garlic's ability to lower cholesterol levels, reduce blood pressure, and improve cardiovascular health. Other research has explored garlic's potential in cancer prevention, immune support, and even cognitive function, painting a vivid picture of garlic as a versatile and potent ally in the quest for optimal health.

As we navigate the intricate pathways of garlic's biochemical complexity, let us marvel at the elegance of nature's design and the profound impact that this humble herb can have on our well-being. For in the crucible of scientific inquiry, we find not only answers to age-old questions but also the promise of new discoveries—and the enduring legacy of garlic as a beacon of hope in the quest for health and vitality.

Sources:
- Amagase, Harunobu, et al. "Intake of Garlic and Its Bioactive Components." The Journal of Nutrition, vol. 131, no. 3, 2001, pp. 955S–962S.
- Lawson, Larry D., and Wallace B. Hughes. "Human absorption of garlic oil constituents: validation of a human in vitro model." Nutrition Research, vol. 16, no. 2, 1996, pp. 245–254.
- Tattelman, Ellen. "Health effects of garlic." American Family Physician, vol. 72, no. 1, 2005, pp. 103–106.

Chapter 5: Garlic's Role in Traditional Medicine Systems

In traditional medicine, garlic stands as a revered and ubiquitous remedy—a potent medicine that has been prized for millennia for its remarkable healing properties. Join me now as we embark on a journey through the diverse tapestry of traditional healing practices, where garlic emerges as a cornerstone of health and wellness across cultures and continents.

Examination of Garlic's Use in Traditional Healing Practices Worldwide
From the sun-baked plains of Africa to the mist-shrouded mountains of Asia, garlic has been embraced by traditional healers as a panacea for a wide range of ailments. In the ancient healing systems of Ayurveda, garlic is known as "**Rasona**," revered for its ability to balance the doshas and promote overall well-being. In traditional African medicine, garlic is used to treat everything from infections to infertility, its pungent aroma believed to drive away evil spirits and negative energy.

Comparison of Garlic's Medicinal Applications in Ayurveda, Traditional Chinese Medicine, and Other Systems
While the specific uses of garlic may vary from one traditional medicine system to another, certain themes and patterns emerge across cultures. In Traditional Chinese Medicine, garlic is prized for its ability to dispel dampness and phlegm, making it a valuable remedy for respiratory ailments and digestive disorders. Similarly, in the indigenous healing traditions of the Americas, garlic

is used to support immune function and ward off infectious diseases, reflecting a universal recognition of its therapeutic potential.

Traditional Remedies and Preparations Featuring Garlic
In the hands of traditional healers, garlic takes on many forms—from teas and tinctures to poultices and potions. In Ayurveda, garlic is often combined with other herbs and spices to create potent remedies for specific health conditions, while in Traditional Chinese Medicine, it may be simmered in soups or stir-fries to enhance its medicinal properties. Across cultures, garlic is revered not only for its efficacy but also for its accessibility, making it a cherished ally in the quest for health and vitality.

Cultural Perspectives on Garlic's Healing Properties
Beyond its physical healing properties, garlic holds a deep cultural significance for many communities around the world. In some cultures, garlic is believed to possess spiritual qualities, serving as a symbol of protection and purity. In others, it is celebrated as a culinary staple, woven into the fabric of everyday life through traditional dishes and festive celebrations. Yet, across cultures, one thing remains constant: the enduring reverence for garlic as a source of strength, resilience, and well-being.

As we explore the rich tapestry of garlic's role in traditional medicine systems, let us honor the wisdom of our ancestors and thank God for the timeless legacy of this remarkable herb. For in the pages of history, we find not only remedies for the body but also nourishment for the soul—a reminder of the profound interconnectedness of humanity and the natural world.

Sources:
- Frawley, David, and Vasant Lad. The Yoga of Herbs: An Ayurvedic Guide to Herbal Medicine. Lotus Press, 2001.
- Tierra, Michael. The Way of Herbs: Fully Updated with the Latest Developments in Herbal Science. Pocket Books, 1980.
- Wang, Tao, et al. "Traditional Chinese Medicine and its role in treatment of osteoarthritis." Journal of Traditional Chinese Medicine, vol. 33, no. 1, 2013, pp. 55–59.

Chapter 6: Cultivating Garlic: From Soil to Plate

In the interaction between earth and sun, water and air, garlic thrives as a testament to the enduring rhythms of nature. Join me now as we embark on a journey into the heart of garlic cultivation, where the simple act of planting a bulb becomes a celebration of life, sustenance, and the timeless cycle of growth and renewal.

Introduction to Garlic Cultivation Techniques
Garlic cultivation is an art as ancient as civilization itself, passed down through generations of farmers and gardeners who have tended to this humble herb with care and reverence. Whether in backyard gardens or vast agricultural fields, the principles of garlic cultivation remain the same: patience, diligence, and a deep respect for the rhythms of nature.

Selection of Suitable Garlic Varieties for Different Climates
One of the keys to successful garlic cultivation lies in the selection of suitable varieties for your climate and growing conditions. From the rich, loamy soils of the Midwest to the sandy coastal plains of the Mediterranean, garlic adapts itself to a wide range of environments, each with its own unique challenges and opportunities. By choosing varieties that are well-suited to your local climate, you can ensure a bountiful harvest of plump, flavorful bulbs.

Soil Preparation, Planting, and Maintenance Tips
Like any garden crop, garlic thrives in well-drained, fertile soil that is rich in organic matter. Before planting, it is essential to prepare the soil by incorporating compost or aged manure to improve its texture and fertility. Garlic cloves should be planted in the fall, several weeks before the first frost, to allow for proper root development before winter sets in. Once planted, garlic requires minimal maintenance, with occasional watering and mulching to suppress weeds and conserve soil moisture.

Harvesting, Curing, and Storing Garlic Bulbs
As the days grow longer and the sun climbs higher in the sky, garlic plants begin to send up tall, slender stalks adorned with fragrant white flowers. This is the signal that it is time to harvest your garlic bulbs, typically in late spring or early summer. To ensure optimal flavor and storage life, it is important to harvest garlic bulbs when the foliage has begun to yellow and dry, but before it has completely withered. Once harvested, garlic bulbs should be cured in a warm, dry place for several weeks to allow them to develop their characteristic flavor and aroma. Once cured, garlic bulbs can be stored in a cool, dry place for several months, providing a steady supply of this culinary treasure throughout the year.

As we dig our hands into the rich, fertile soil and watch with wonder as garlic bulbs take root and grow, let us savor the simple pleasures of cultivating our own food—a reminder of our deep connection to the land and the nourishing bounty it provides.

25

Sources:
- Meredith, Ted. The Complete Book of Garlic: A Guide for Gardeners, Growers, and Serious Cooks. Timber Press, 2008.
- Rees, Ailsa. The Garlic Farm Cookbook: Recipes and Tips from the King of Garlic. Ryland Peters & Small, 2015.
- Stout, Ruth, and David Cavagnaro. Growing Great Garlic: The Definitive Guide for Organic Gardeners and Small Farmers. Chelsea Green Publishing, 1991.

Chapter 7: Exploring the Varieties of Garlic: A World of Flavors

Step into the amazing world of garlic varieties, where each bulb tells a story of soil, climate, and centuries-old traditions. Come with me as we embark on a culinary journey across continents and cultures, exploring the diverse array of flavors, aromas, and textures that make garlic a true treasure of the earth.

Overview of the Wide Range of Garlic Cultivars
From the fiery heat of Rocambole to the mellow sweetness of Elephant garlic, the world of garlic cultivars is as vast and varied as the landscapes from which they hail. With thousands of varieties to choose from, each with its own unique characteristics, garlic enthusiasts are spoiled for choice when it comes to selecting the perfect bulbs for their garden or kitchen.

Distinctive Flavor Profiles and Characteristics of Different Garlic Varieties
No two garlic varieties are alike, and each offers its own distinctive flavor profile and culinary potential. Softneck varieties, such as California Early and Italian Purple, are prized for their mild, sweet flavor and long shelf life, making them ideal for braiding and storage. Hardneck varieties, such as German Red and Chesnok Red, boast a more robust flavor and are well-suited to roasting, grilling, and other high-heat cooking methods.

Regional Specialties and Heirloom Varieties
In every corner of the globe, garlic has taken on unique characteristics shaped by the soil, climate, and cultural traditions of its native region. From the pungent Purple

Stripe varieties of Eastern Europe to the delicate Silverskin varieties of California, each garlic cultivar tells a story of place and people—a living testament to the rich tapestry of human experience.

Tips for Selecting the Right Garlic for Culinary and Medicinal Use
When selecting garlic for culinary or medicinal use, it is important to consider not only its flavor and aroma but also its intended application. Softneck varieties are well-suited to raw applications, such as salads and dressings, while hardneck varieties excel when cooked, imparting their rich, complex flavors to soups, stews, and sauces. For medicinal use, it is important to choose garlic varieties that are high in allicin and other beneficial compounds, ensuring maximum potency and efficacy.

As we explore the vast and varied world of garlic varieties, let us celebrate the diversity of flavors, aromas, and textures that make this humble herb a true culinary treasure. Whether grown in backyard gardens or harvested from far-flung fields, each bulb of garlic offers a glimpse into the rich tapestry of human culture and the enduring bond between food and community.

Sources:
- Block, Eric. Garlic and Other Alliums: The Lore and the Science. Royal Society of Chemistry, 2010.
- Engeland, Ellen. The Garlic Papers: A Small Garlic Cookbook. William Morrow & Co, 1981.
- Rowles, Linda. The Essential Garlic Cookbook. Lorenz Books, 1997.

Chapter 8: Garlic in Culinary Traditions Around the Globe

Psych up your taste buds for a tantalizing journey across continents and cultures as we explore the ubiquitous presence of garlic in cuisines from around the world. From the fiery kitchens of Asia to the rustic trattorias of Italy, garlic weaves its magic into a tapestry of flavors, aromas, and culinary traditions that delight the senses and nourish the soul.

Survey of Garlic's Prominent Role in Global Cuisines
Garlic transcends borders and boundaries, taking center stage in a diverse array of culinary traditions from every corner of the globe. In Mediterranean cuisine, garlic is a foundational ingredient, lending its pungent aroma and robust flavor to everything from pasta sauces to seafood dishes. In Asian cuisines, garlic is prized for its ability to add depth and complexity to stir-fries, curries, and noodle dishes, while in Latin America, it is celebrated for its role in salsas, marinades, and stews.

Signature Garlic Dishes from Various Cultures
Every culture has its iconic garlic dishes, beloved for their bold flavors and timeless appeal. In France, garlic takes center stage in the classic dish, Chicken with 40 Cloves of Garlic, where whole cloves are roasted until golden and caramelized, infusing the meat with their rich, mellow flavor. In Korea, garlic shines in the fiery-sweet marinade of Bulgogi, where thinly sliced beef is bathed in a mixture of soy sauce, sugar, and minced garlic before being grilled to perfection. And in Italy, garlic lends its unmistakable aroma to the hearty bean soup known as Pasta e Fagioli, where it mingles

with tomatoes, herbs, and creamy cannellini beans to create a dish that is as comforting as it is satisfying.

Culinary Techniques for Maximizing Garlic Flavor
To unlock the full potential of garlic's flavor, it is essential to master a few simple culinary techniques. Whether sautéing, roasting, or grilling, the key lies in controlling the temperature and cooking time to achieve the perfect balance of sweetness, richness, and depth. For raw applications, such as salads and dressings, garlic should be finely minced or grated to release its potent aroma and flavor. And for dishes where a milder, sweeter flavor is desired, garlic can be roasted whole until soft and caramelized, imparting a subtle sweetness to the finished dish.

Creative Ways to Incorporate Garlic into Everyday Cooking
Beyond its traditional uses, garlic offers endless possibilities for creative culinary expression. From garlic-infused oils and vinegars to garlic-flavored salts and spreads, the options are limited only by your imagination. Try adding roasted garlic to mashed potatoes for a creamy, decadent side dish, or toss whole cloves with olive oil and herbs for a simple yet elegant appetizer. And don't forget about garlic's versatility as a flavor enhancer in soups, salads, and sauces—wherever you go, garlic is sure to add a touch of magic to every meal.

As we savor the rich and varied flavors of garlic in cuisines from around the world, let us celebrate the timeless appeal of this humble herb and the culinary traditions that have shaped it into the beloved ingredient it is today. For in the kitchen, as in life, garlic has the power to transform the ordinary into the extraordinary, one clove at a time.

Sources:
- Davidson, Alan. The Oxford Companion to Food. Oxford University Press, 2014.
- Ottolenghi, Yotam, and Sami Tamimi. Jerusalem: A Cookbook. Ten Speed Press, 2012.
- Sandler, Linda. The Garlic Cookbook. HP Books, 1992.

Chapter 9: Garlic's Nutritional Profile: A Closer Look

In the realm of nutrition, garlic emerges as a true powerhouse—a humble herb that packs a punch when it comes to vitamins, minerals, and antioxidants. Join me now as we peel back the layers of this culinary treasure to uncover the wealth of nutrients that lie within, and explore the myriad ways in which garlic can support our health and well-being.

Nutritional Composition of Garlic Bulbs
At its core, garlic is a nutritional powerhouse, rich in essential vitamins, minerals, and bioactive compounds that nourish the body and invigorate the soul. A single clove of garlic contains a wealth of nutrients, including vitamin C, vitamin B6, manganese, and selenium, as well as trace amounts of calcium, potassium, and iron. Low in calories and fat, yet high in flavor and aroma, garlic is a true gem of the culinary world.

Vitamins, Minerals, and Antioxidants Found in Garlic
Garlic's nutritional bounty extends far beyond its basic vitamins and minerals, encompassing a diverse array of antioxidants and phytochemicals that contribute to its health-promoting properties. Allicin, the compound responsible for garlic's distinctive odor, is not only a potent antimicrobial agent but also a powerful antioxidant that helps neutralize harmful free radicals in the body. Other sulfur-containing compounds in garlic, such as diallyl sulfides and ajoene, have been shown to possess anti-inflammatory, anticancer, and cardiovascular benefits, making garlic a true superfood for the ages.

Health Implications of Garlic's Nutritional Content
The nutritional content of garlic has profound implications for health and wellness, with research suggesting that regular consumption of garlic may help reduce the risk of chronic diseases such as heart disease, cancer, and diabetes. Garlic's antioxidant properties help protect against oxidative stress and inflammation, while its ability to lower cholesterol and blood pressure levels supports cardiovascular health. Additionally, garlic's antimicrobial effects make it a valuable ally in the fight against infections and immune-related disorders.

Recommended Dietary Intake of Garlic for Optimal Health
While there is no one-size-fits-all recommendation for garlic intake, incorporating garlic into your daily diet can offer a wide range of health benefits. Whether consumed raw, cooked, or in supplement form, garlic can be enjoyed in moderation as part of a balanced diet rich in fruits, vegetables, whole grains, and lean proteins. For optimal health benefits, aim to include garlic in your meals several times per week, and experiment with different culinary techniques to maximize its flavor and nutritional content.

As we celebrate the nutritional riches of garlic, let us savor the simple pleasure of nourishing our bodies with nature's bounty—a reminder of the profound impact that food can have on our health and well-being. For in the vibrant hues of a garlic bulb, we find not only sustenance for the body but also nourishment for the soul—a testament to the enduring power of food as medicine.

Sources:

- Gardner, Amanda, et al. "A systematic review of garlic consumption and cancer risk." American Journal of Clinical Nutrition, vol. 104, no. 4, 2016, pp. 1027–1039.
- Rahman, Khalid, and Fazal-ur-Rehman Bhatti. "Garlic (Allium sativum): a review of its adverse effects on health." Journal of Toxicology and Environmental Health Sciences, vol. 4, no. 1, 2012, pp. 1–6.
- Ried, Karin, et al. "The effect of garlic on cholesterol and blood pressure: a systematic review and meta-analysis." Nutrition Reviews, vol. 71, no. 5, 2013, pp. 282–299.

Chapter 10: Harnessing the Allicin: Garlic's Key Compound

Prepare to unlock the secrets of garlic's most potent compound as we delve deep into the world of allicin—a powerhouse of health and vitality. Join me as we explore the remarkable properties, benefits, and therapeutic potential of allicin, and discover the myriad ways in which this humble compound can transform our health and well-being.

In-Depth Exploration of Allicin's Properties and Benefits
At the heart of garlic's medicinal prowess lies allicin, a sulfur-containing compound that is formed when garlic cloves are crushed or chopped. Allicin is responsible for garlic's distinctive aroma and flavor, as well as many of its health-promoting properties. As a natural antimicrobial agent, allicin helps fight infections, while its antioxidant properties help protect against oxidative stress and inflammation. Additionally, allicin has been shown to support cardiovascular health, lower cholesterol levels, and even inhibit the growth of cancer cells—an impressive array of benefits for a single compound.

Factors Influencing Allicin Formation in Garlic
The formation of allicin in garlic is a complex process influenced by a variety of factors, including the age, variety, and storage conditions of the garlic bulbs. Young garlic bulbs tend to contain higher levels of allicin precursors, while older bulbs may have lower concentrations due to enzymatic breakdown over time. Additionally, allicin formation is enhanced by crushing

or chopping garlic cloves, which releases the enzyme alliinase and allows it to convert alliin into allicin—a process that occurs within seconds of exposure to air.

Methods for Preserving Allicin Content in Garlic Preparations
To maximize the allicin content in garlic preparations, it is important to handle garlic with care and precision. Crushing or chopping garlic cloves immediately before use ensures the highest levels of allicin formation, while prolonged storage or exposure to heat can cause allicin to degrade over time. To preserve allicin content in garlic supplements or extracts, manufacturers may use techniques such as freeze-drying or low-temperature processing, which help retain the compound's potency and efficacy.

Health Effects of Allicin and Its Potential Therapeutic Applications
The health effects of allicin are far-reaching, with research suggesting that this powerful compound may offer therapeutic benefits for a wide range of conditions. In addition to its antimicrobial and antioxidant properties, allicin has been shown to support immune function, improve cardiovascular health, and even protect against certain types of cancer. As a natural remedy with few side effects, allicin holds great promise as a complementary therapy for individuals seeking to optimize their health and well-being.

As we unravel the mysteries of allicin and its profound impact on human health, let us celebrate the remarkable synergy between nature and science—a testament to the enduring power of garlic as a source of healing and vitality.

Sources:

- Ankri, Serge, and David Mirelman. "Antimicrobial properties of allicin from garlic." Microbes and Infection, vol. 1, no. 2, 1999, pp. 125–129.
- Lawson, Larry D., and Wallace B. Hughes. "Absorption of allicin from garlic." Planta Medica, vol. 60, no. 04, 1994, pp. 355–357.
- Sivam, Ganesan P. "Protection against Helicobacter pylori and other bacterial infections by garlic." Journal of Nutrition, vol. 131, no. 3, 2001, pp. 1106S–1108S.

Chapter 11: Garlic's Antimicrobial Properties: Fighting Infections Naturally

Prepare to embark on a journey into the realm of natural healing as we explore the remarkable antimicrobial properties of garlic—a potent ally in the fight against bacterial, fungal, and viral infections. Join me as we unravel the mechanisms by which garlic combats pathogens, delve into the scientific evidence supporting its effectiveness, and discover practical applications for harnessing garlic's healing power in preventing and treating infections.

Overview of Garlic's Antimicrobial Properties
Garlic has long been revered for its ability to fend off microbial invaders, earning it a rightful place in the pantheon of natural remedies. From ancient civilizations to modern laboratories, garlic has been celebrated for its potent antimicrobial properties, which encompass a wide range of pathogens, including bacteria, fungi, and viruses. At the heart of garlic's antimicrobial prowess lies allicin, a sulfur-containing compound that acts as nature's own antibiotic, targeting and neutralizing harmful microorganisms with remarkable precision.

Mechanisms by Which Garlic Combats Bacterial, Fungal, and Viral Infections
The mechanisms by which garlic combats infections are as diverse as the pathogens themselves, with garlic employing a multi-faceted approach to microbial warfare. Allicin, garlic's primary active ingredient, disrupts the integrity of bacterial cell membranes, inhibiting their growth and replication. Additionally, garlic's sulfur-containing compounds interfere with the

metabolic processes of fungi, disrupting their ability to thrive and spread. When it comes to viral infections, garlic's immune-boosting properties help strengthen the body's natural defenses, making it more resistant to viral invaders and speeding up the recovery process.

Scientific Evidence Supporting Garlic's Effectiveness as a Natural Antimicrobial Agent
Decades of scientific research have provided compelling evidence of garlic's effectiveness as a natural antimicrobial agent, with numerous studies demonstrating its ability to inhibit the growth of a wide range of pathogens. Clinical trials have shown that garlic supplements can help reduce the severity and duration of respiratory infections, while laboratory studies have revealed garlic's ability to kill antibiotic-resistant bacteria and combat fungal infections such as candida. With its broad spectrum of activity and minimal side effects, garlic offers a safe and effective alternative to conventional antimicrobial agents.

Practical Applications of Garlic for Preventing and Treating Infections
Incorporating garlic into your daily routine is a simple yet powerful way to bolster your body's defenses against infections. Whether consumed raw, cooked, or in supplement form, garlic can be a valuable ally in preventing and treating a variety of ailments, from the common cold to more serious infections. For optimal effectiveness, aim to include garlic in your meals regularly, and consider using garlic supplements during cold and flu season or when traveling to areas where infectious diseases are prevalent.

As we harness the antimicrobial power of garlic to fight infections naturally, let us celebrate the remarkable synergy between science and nature—a testament to the enduring wisdom of traditional healing practices and the boundless potential of the natural world.

Sources:
- Ankri, Serge, and David Mirelman. "Antimicrobial properties of allicin from garlic." Microbes and Infection, vol. 1, no. 2, 1999, pp. 125–129.
- Harris, John C., et al. "Ajoene inhibits both primary tumor growth and metastasis of B16F10 melanoma cells in C57BL/6 mice." Cancer Letters, vol. 101, no. 2, 1996, pp. 199–205.
- Reiter, Markus, and Hans-Jörg Brandt. "Rapid detection of allicin in garlic: Use of a gas sensor optimized by experimental design." Journal of Agricultural and Food Chemistry, vol. 55, no. 2, 2007, pp. 536–540.

Chapter 12: Garlic for Heart Health: Lowering Cholesterol and Blood Pressure

Prepare to delve into the realm of cardiovascular wellness as we uncover the remarkable benefits of garlic for heart health. Join me on a journey through the intricate pathways of cholesterol metabolism and blood pressure regulation, and discover how garlic, nature's own elixir, can help safeguard your cardiovascular system and promote a lifetime of heart health.

Explanation of Garlic's Cardiovascular Benefits
Garlic has long been revered for its ability to promote cardiovascular health, earning it a well-deserved place in the pantheon of natural remedies. From ancient healers to modern physicians, garlic has been celebrated for its ability to lower cholesterol levels, reduce blood pressure, and support overall heart function. At the heart of garlic's cardiovascular benefits lies its rich array of bioactive compounds, including allicin, which work synergistically to protect against heart disease and stroke.

Impact of Garlic on Cholesterol Levels and Lipid Profiles
High cholesterol levels are a major risk factor for heart disease, making it essential to maintain healthy lipid profiles to reduce the risk of cardiovascular events. Garlic has been shown to exert beneficial effects on cholesterol levels by lowering total cholesterol, LDL ("bad") cholesterol, and triglycerides, while increasing HDL ("good") cholesterol—the protective lipid that helps clear cholesterol from the bloodstream. By modulating lipid metabolism and inhibiting cholesterol synthesis, garlic helps promote a healthy balance of fats

in the blood, reducing the risk of atherosclerosis and coronary artery disease.

Mechanisms of Action Behind Garlic's Ability to Lower Blood Pressure

Hypertension, or high blood pressure, is another key risk factor for heart disease, affecting millions of people worldwide. Garlic has been shown to exert blood pressure-lowering effects through multiple mechanisms, including vasodilation, inhibition of angiotensin-converting enzyme (ACE), and reduction of oxidative stress and inflammation. By relaxing blood vessels and improving blood flow, garlic helps lower blood pressure levels, reducing the strain on the heart and lowering the risk of cardiovascular complications.

Clinical Studies Assessing Garlic's Efficacy in Promoting Heart Health

Decades of clinical research have provided compelling evidence of garlic's efficacy in promoting heart health, with numerous studies demonstrating its ability to lower cholesterol levels, reduce blood pressure, and improve overall cardiovascular function. Meta-analyses of randomized controlled trials have confirmed the beneficial effects of garlic supplementation on lipid profiles and blood pressure, suggesting that garlic may offer a safe and effective adjunctive therapy for individuals at risk of heart disease.

As we embrace the cardiovascular benefits of garlic, let us celebrate the power of nature to heal and protect our most vital organ—the heart. For in the fragrant cloves of garlic, we find not only the promise of a healthier future but also the timeless wisdom of traditional medicine and the boundless potential of the natural world.

Sources:
- Ried, Karin, et al. "The effect of garlic on cholesterol and blood pressure: a systematic review and meta-analysis." Nutrition Reviews, vol. 71, no. 5, 2013, pp. 282–299.
- Sobenin, Igor A., et al. "The effects of time-released garlic powder tablets on multifunctional cardiovascular risk in patients with coronary artery disease." Lipids in Health and Disease, vol. 17, no. 1, 2018, p. 178.
- Steiner, M., et al. "A double-blind crossover study in moderately hypercholesterolemic men that compared the effect of aged garlic extract and placebo administration on blood lipids." American Journal of Clinical Nutrition, vol. 64, no. 6, 1996, pp. 866–870.

Chapter 13: Garlic and Cancer Prevention: Separating Fact from Fiction

In the quest for cancer prevention, garlic emerges as a subject of both curiosity and contention. Join me now as we embark on a journey through the labyrinth of scientific research, separating fact from fiction to uncover the truth about garlic's potential role in cancer prevention. From laboratory studies to clinical trials, we'll explore the evidence, mechanisms, and recommendations for incorporating garlic into a cancer-preventive lifestyle.

Examination of Garlic's Potential Role in Cancer Prevention
For centuries, garlic has been celebrated for its medicinal properties, including its purported ability to prevent cancer. While anecdotal evidence and traditional wisdom abound, scientific research has yielded mixed results, leaving many questions unanswered. As we navigate the complex landscape of cancer prevention, it is essential to critically examine the evidence and weigh the potential benefits of garlic against its limitations.

Overview of Studies Investigating Garlic's Effects on Various Types of Cancer
Over the years, numerous studies have sought to elucidate the relationship between garlic consumption and cancer risk, with varying degrees of success. While some studies have reported a protective effect of garlic against certain types of cancer, such as gastric, colorectal, and prostate cancer, others have found no significant association or even an increased risk in some

cases. As researchers continue to unravel the complexities of cancer biology, the role of garlic in cancer prevention remains a topic of ongoing debate and investigation.

Possible Mechanisms by Which Garlic May Inhibit Carcinogenesis

The mechanisms by which garlic may inhibit carcinogenesis are multifaceted and complex, involving a combination of antioxidant, anti-inflammatory, and immunomodulatory effects. Garlic's rich array of bioactive compounds, including allicin, diallyl sulfide, and S-allyl cysteine, have been shown to interfere with various stages of cancer development, including tumor initiation, promotion, and progression. By scavenging free radicals, suppressing inflammatory pathways, and enhancing immune surveillance, garlic may help protect against DNA damage, cell proliferation, and tumor formation.

Recommendations for Incorporating Garlic into a Cancer-Preventive Lifestyle

While the evidence supporting garlic's role in cancer prevention remains inconclusive, incorporating garlic into a balanced, plant-based diet may offer additional health benefits beyond cancer risk reduction. Garlic's antioxidant and anti-inflammatory properties, combined with its ability to support cardiovascular health and immune function, make it a valuable addition to a cancer-preventive lifestyle. To maximize the potential benefits of garlic, aim to include fresh garlic in your meals regularly, and consider incorporating garlic supplements into your daily routine for added support.

As we navigate the complex terrain of cancer prevention, let us approach garlic with both curiosity and caution, recognizing its potential as a complementary strategy for reducing cancer risk while acknowledging the limitations of current scientific evidence. For in the pursuit of health and well-being, knowledge is our most powerful ally, guiding us on a journey of discovery and empowerment.

Sources:
- Fleischauer, Aaron T., et al. "Garlic consumption and cancer prevention: meta-analyses of colorectal and stomach cancers." American Journal of Clinical Nutrition, vol. 72, no. 4, 2000, pp. 1047–1052.
- Kim, J-S., and E. G. Lee. "Anti-cancer effects of garlic-derived compounds in cancer." Journal of Medicinal Food, vol. 7, no. 3, 2004, pp. 327–341.
- Powolny, Anna A., and Shivendra V. Singh. "Multitargeted prevention and therapy of cancer by diallyl trisulfide and related Allium vegetable-derived organosulfur compounds." Cancer Letters, vol. 269, no. 2, 2008, pp. 305–314.

Chapter 14: Digestive Wellness: Soothing the Gut Naturally

Embark on a journey to unlock the secrets of digestive wellness as we explore the remarkable benefits of garlic for nurturing a healthy gut. Join me as we delve into the digestive benefits of garlic, uncover its role in promoting gut health, and discover practical tips for harnessing garlic's soothing properties to alleviate digestive issues and restore balance to your inner ecosystem.

Discussion of Garlic's Digestive Benefits
Garlic, celebrated for its culinary prowess and medicinal properties, offers a wealth of benefits for digestive wellness. From soothing upset stomachs to promoting optimal digestion, garlic has earned its place as a cherished ally in the quest for gut health. Whether consumed raw, cooked, or in supplement form, garlic's rich array of bioactive compounds, including allicin and diallyl sulfides, work synergistically to support the digestive process and nourish the gut microbiota.

How Garlic Promotes Digestive Health and Aids in Digestion
Garlic aids digestion through multiple mechanisms, beginning with its ability to stimulate the production of digestive enzymes and gastric juices, which help break down food and facilitate nutrient absorption. Additionally, garlic's anti-inflammatory and antimicrobial properties help soothe irritated tissues, reduce bloating and gas, and promote regularity—a boon for individuals struggling with digestive discomfort. By supporting healthy digestion and gut motility, garlic helps maintain balance and harmony

within the digestive system, promoting overall wellness and vitality.

Garlic's Role in Supporting Gut Microbiota Balance
The gut microbiota, a complex ecosystem of microorganisms that inhabit the digestive tract, plays a crucial role in digestive health, immune function, and overall well-being. Garlic, with its prebiotic properties and antimicrobial effects, helps support a diverse and resilient gut microbiota by nourishing beneficial bacteria and inhibiting the growth of harmful pathogens. By fostering a healthy balance of gut microbes, garlic helps maintain optimal digestion, nutrient absorption, and immune function, reducing the risk of digestive disorders and promoting long-term wellness.

Practical Tips for Using Garlic to Alleviate Digestive Issues
Incorporating garlic into your daily routine is a simple yet effective way to support digestive wellness and alleviate common gastrointestinal complaints. Whether added to soups, stews, salads, or stir-fries, garlic infuses dishes with its aromatic flavor and soothing properties, promoting optimal digestion and gut health. For individuals with sensitive stomachs, cooked garlic may be easier to tolerate than raw garlic, while garlic supplements offer a convenient option for those seeking targeted digestive support. Experiment with different culinary techniques and recipes to find creative ways to incorporate garlic into your meals, and listen to your body's cues to determine what works best for you.

As we embrace the digestive benefits of garlic, let us savor the simple pleasure of nourishing our bodies with nature's bounty—a reminder of the profound connection between food and health, and the power of garlic to heal and restore balance to our inner ecosystem.

Sources:
- McFarland, Lynne V. "Use of probiotics to correct dysbiosis of normal microbiota following disease or disruptive events: a systematic review." BMJ Open, vol. 4, no. 8, 2014, e005047.
- Rees, Karen, et al. "Garlic for preventing cardiovascular events." Cochrane Database of Systematic Reviews, vol. 8, 2012, CD006095.
- Ried, Karin, et al. "The effect of garlic on cholesterol and blood pressure: a systematic review and meta-analysis." Nutrition Reviews, vol. 71, no. 5, 2013, pp. 282–299.

Chapter 15: Garlic's Immune-Boosting Abilities: Shielding Against Illness

Prepare to fortify your body's natural defenses as we uncover the immune-boosting powers of garlic—a humble herb with extraordinary potential to shield against illness and infection. Join me on a journey through the intricate pathways of the immune system, as we explore garlic's immune-enhancing properties, mechanisms of action, and evidence from studies demonstrating its ability to prevent and alleviate colds, flu, and other infections. Armed with knowledge and insight, we'll discover practical strategies for incorporating garlic into your daily routine to strengthen your immune system and safeguard your health.

Exploration of Garlic's Immune-Enhancing Properties
Garlic has long been revered for its medicinal properties, including its ability to bolster the immune system and fend off illness. From ancient civilizations to modern science, garlic has been celebrated for its potent immune-enhancing properties, which stem from its rich array of bioactive compounds, including allicin, diallyl sulfides, and S-allyl cysteine. As we delve deeper into the realm of immune health, we'll uncover the secrets of garlic's immune-boosting abilities and their profound implications for overall well-being.

How Garlic Boosts the Immune System's Defense Mechanisms
Garlic supports immune function through multiple mechanisms, acting as a natural immunomodulator that helps regulate and optimize the body's immune response. By stimulating the production and activity of

immune cells, such as macrophages, T cells, and natural killer cells, garlic enhances the body's ability to recognize and neutralize foreign invaders, including bacteria, viruses, and other pathogens. Additionally, garlic's antioxidant and anti-inflammatory properties help protect against oxidative stress and inflammation, which can compromise immune function and increase susceptibility to infection.

Evidence from Studies on Garlic's Ability to Prevent and Alleviate Infections
Numerous studies have investigated the role of garlic in preventing and alleviating infections, with promising results supporting its immune-boosting effects. Clinical trials have demonstrated that garlic supplementation can help reduce the frequency, severity, and duration of colds and flu, as well as other respiratory infections. Additionally, laboratory studies have shown that garlic exhibits broad-spectrum antimicrobial activity against a wide range of pathogens, making it a valuable ally in the fight against infectious diseases.

Strategies for Using Garlic to Strengthen the Immune System
Incorporating garlic into your daily routine is a simple yet powerful way to strengthen your immune system and protect against illness. Whether consumed raw, cooked, or in supplement form, garlic offers a versatile and convenient option for immune support. To maximize its benefits, aim to include garlic in your meals regularly, and consider adding garlic supplements to your daily regimen during cold and flu season or when traveling to areas where infectious diseases are prevalent. Additionally, experiment with garlic-rich

recipes and culinary techniques to explore the full range of flavors and aromas that garlic has to offer.

As we harness the immune-boosting powers of garlic to shield against illness and infection, let us embrace the wisdom of nature and the boundless potential of this humble herb to nourish, protect, and heal.

Sources:
- Josling, Peter. "Preventing the common cold with a garlic supplement: a double-blind, placebo-controlled survey." Advances in Therapy, vol. 18, no. 4, 2001, pp. 189–193.
- Nantz, Meri P., et al. "Supplementation with aged garlic extract improves both NK and γδ-T cell function and reduces the severity of cold and flu symptoms: a randomized, double-blind, placebo-controlled nutrition intervention." Clinical Nutrition, vol. 31, no. 3, 2012, pp. 337–344.
- Percival, Susan S. "Aged garlic extract modifies human immunity." Journal of Nutrition, vol. 146, no. 2, 2016, pp. 433S–436S.

Chapter 16: Garlic for Respiratory Health: Easing Symptoms Naturally

Get ready to breathe easier as we explore the extraordinary benefits of garlic for respiratory wellness—a natural remedy with the power to soothe, strengthen, and support the lungs. Join me on a journey through the intricate pathways of respiratory health, as we uncover garlic's ability to alleviate symptoms of respiratory infections, allergies, and asthma, backed by scientific evidence and practical insights into incorporating garlic into your daily routine for optimal lung function and vitality.

Overview of Garlic's Benefits for Respiratory Wellness
Garlic has long been revered for its medicinal properties, including its ability to promote respiratory health and ease symptoms of common respiratory ailments. From ancient healers to modern physicians, garlic has been celebrated for its potent anti-inflammatory, antimicrobial, and immune-boosting properties, which make it a valuable ally in the fight against respiratory infections, allergies, and asthma. As we embark on a journey to explore garlic's respiratory benefits, we'll uncover the secrets of this humble herb and its profound implications for lung health and vitality.

How Garlic Helps Alleviate Symptoms of Respiratory Infections, Allergies, and Asthma
Garlic offers a multifaceted approach to respiratory wellness, addressing the underlying causes of respiratory ailments while providing relief from symptoms. Whether combating viral and bacterial infections or soothing inflammation and irritation,

garlic's rich array of bioactive compounds, including allicin and quercetin, work synergistically to promote lung health and function. By boosting immune function, reducing inflammation, and inhibiting the growth of pathogens, garlic helps alleviate symptoms of respiratory infections, while its anti-inflammatory properties offer relief from allergies and asthma.

Scientific Evidence Supporting Garlic's Efficacy in Improving Lung Function

Clinical studies have provided compelling evidence of garlic's efficacy in improving lung function and alleviating symptoms of respiratory ailments. Research has shown that garlic supplementation can help reduce the frequency, severity, and duration of respiratory infections, as well as improve lung function in individuals with asthma and chronic obstructive pulmonary disease (COPD). Additionally, laboratory studies have demonstrated garlic's ability to inhibit airway inflammation and bronchoconstriction, suggesting its potential as a complementary therapy for respiratory conditions.

Practical Ways to Incorporate Garlic into Respiratory Health Routines

Incorporating garlic into your daily routine is a simple yet effective way to support respiratory health and alleviate symptoms of respiratory ailments. Whether consumed raw, cooked, or in supplement form, garlic offers a versatile and convenient option for respiratory support. To maximize its benefits, aim to include garlic in your meals regularly, and consider adding garlic supplements to your daily regimen during cold and flu season or when experiencing respiratory symptoms.

Additionally, experiment with garlic-rich recipes and culinary techniques to explore the full range of flavors and aromas that garlic has to offer.

As we embrace the respiratory benefits of garlic, let us breathe easier knowing that nature has provided us with a powerful ally in the quest for lung health and vitality.

Sources:
- Josling, Peter. "Preventing the common cold with a garlic supplement: a double-blind, placebo-controlled survey." Advances in Therapy, vol. 18, no. 4, 2001, pp. 189–193.
- Larijani, Bagher, et al. "The efficacy of adjunctive therapy with garlic in primary isolated coronary artery bypass graft patients with high blood lipid levels: a randomized controlled clinical trial." Nutrition, vol. 32, no. 3, 2016, pp. 276–282.
- Percival, Susan S. "Aged garlic extract modifies human immunity." Journal of Nutrition, vol. 146, no. 2, 2016, pp. 433S–436S.

Chapter 17: Garlic for Skin and Hair: Unlocking Beauty from Within

Stand ready to unveil the secrets of radiant skin and lustrous hair as we explore the transformative benefits of garlic—a natural elixir for beauty from within. Join me on a journey through the realms of skincare and haircare, as we discover garlic's ability to promote healthy skin by combating acne, aging, and other skin conditions, while nourishing the scalp and stimulating hair growth. Armed with knowledge and practical insights, we'll explore DIY beauty recipes featuring garlic, empowering you to unlock your natural beauty potential and radiate confidence from head to toe.

Explanation of Garlic's Skin and Hair Benefits
Garlic, celebrated for its culinary and medicinal properties, offers a wealth of benefits for skincare and haircare alike. From ancient civilizations to modern beauty rituals, garlic has been revered for its ability to nourish, protect, and rejuvenate the skin and hair. Rich in antioxidants, vitamins, and minerals, garlic promotes healthy skin by combating acne, aging, and other skin conditions, while supporting hair growth and scalp health. As we delve deeper into the beauty-enhancing properties of garlic, we'll uncover the secrets of youthful skin and vibrant hair, waiting to be unlocked.

How Garlic Promotes Healthy Skin by Combating Acne, Aging, and Other Skin Conditions
Garlic's potent antimicrobial, anti-inflammatory, and antioxidant properties make it a valuable ally in the quest for healthy skin. Whether combating acne-causing

bacteria, neutralizing free radicals, or promoting collagen production, garlic addresses the underlying causes of common skin concerns, including acne, wrinkles, and hyperpigmentation. Additionally, garlic's sulfur compounds help regulate sebum production and balance the skin's natural oils, reducing the risk of breakouts and promoting a clear, radiant complexion.

Garlic's Role in Supporting Hair Growth and Scalp Health
Healthy hair begins at the roots, and garlic's nourishing properties extend to the scalp, where it helps promote optimal hair growth and scalp health. Garlic's sulfur compounds, vitamins, and minerals nourish the hair follicles, strengthen the hair shaft, and improve blood circulation to the scalp, stimulating hair growth and preventing hair loss. Additionally, garlic's antimicrobial properties help combat dandruff and other scalp conditions, promoting a healthy scalp environment for vibrant, beautiful hair.

DIY Beauty Recipes Featuring Garlic for Radiant Skin and Lustrous Hair
Experience the transformative power of garlic with DIY beauty recipes that harness its potent properties to enhance your natural beauty. From acne-fighting face masks to hair-strengthening treatments, these simple yet effective recipes offer a natural alternative to commercial skincare and haircare products. Discover the joy of creating your own beauty elixirs using garlic, alongside other nourishing ingredients from nature, and unlock the radiant skin and lustrous hair you've always dreamed of.

As we embrace the beauty-enhancing benefits of garlic, let us celebrate the transformative power of nature to nourish, protect, and rejuvenate our skin and hair. For in the fragrant cloves of garlic, we find not only the promise of radiant beauty but also the timeless wisdom of traditional beauty rituals and the boundless potential of natural ingredients to elevate our self-care routines.

Sources:
- Ali, Badreldin H., and Waseem Ahmed. "Garlic and onions: Their cancer prevention properties." Cancer Causes & Control, vol. 19, no. 1, 2008, pp. 37–44.
- Hasanzade, Farzaneh, et al. "A review of therapeutic effects of garlic (Allium sativum) in dermatology." Dermatology Reports, vol. 10, no. 1, 2018, pp. 7533.
- Rondanelli, Mariangela, et al. "Allium cepa L.: A natural alternative for skin and hair care." Journal of Cosmetics, Dermatological Sciences and Applications, vol. 5, no. 3, 2015, pp. 240–244.

Chapter 18: Garlic as an Aphrodisiac: Love Potion or Myth?

Get set for exploring the tantalizing mysteries of garlic's reputation as an aphrodisiac—a subject steeped in both legend and skepticism. Join me on a journey through the annals of history and culture as we unravel the allure of garlic and its purported effects on libido, examining the scientific evidence (or lack thereof) and considering alternative explanations for garlic's association with romance and desire. Whether myth or reality, the story of garlic as an aphrodisiac offers a fascinating glimpse into the human experience of love, desire, and the quest for intimacy.

Examination of Garlic's Reputation as an Aphrodisiac
Throughout the ages, garlic has captivated the imagination with its potent aroma, distinctive flavor, and enigmatic allure. From ancient civilizations to modern times, garlic has been celebrated for its purported ability to arouse desire and enhance sexual performance—a reputation that has endured across cultures and continents. Yet, amidst the whispers of garlic's aphrodisiac powers, questions linger about the truth behind the myth and the science behind the legend.

Historical and Cultural Beliefs Surrounding Garlic and Its Effects on Libido
Garlic's association with romance and desire can be traced back to ancient times, where it was revered as a symbol of fertility and passion. In cultures around the world, garlic has been incorporated into love potions, wedding rituals, and culinary aphrodisiacs, believed to

ignite the flames of passion and strengthen bonds of intimacy. Whether consumed raw, cooked, or worn as an amulet, garlic has been cherished for its ability to stimulate desire and enhance sexual pleasure—a testament to its enduring legacy as a symbol of love and romance.

Scientific Evidence (or Lack Thereof) Supporting Garlic's Aphrodisiac Properties

While garlic's reputation as an aphrodisiac is deeply ingrained in folklore and tradition, scientific evidence supporting its effects on libido is limited and inconclusive. Despite anecdotal reports and historical accounts, rigorous studies investigating garlic's aphrodisiac properties have yielded mixed results, with some suggesting a potential link between garlic consumption and sexual arousal, while others find no significant association. As researchers continue to explore the complex interplay between diet, lifestyle, and sexual health, the mystery of garlic as an aphrodisiac remains open to interpretation.

Alternative Explanations for Garlic's Association with Romance and Desire

Beyond its purported aphrodisiac properties, garlic's association with romance and desire may be attributed to its symbolic significance and sensory allure. From its pungent aroma to its fiery flavor, garlic tantalizes the senses and evokes feelings of passion and pleasure—a sensory experience that transcends the boundaries of taste and smell. Additionally, garlic's reputation as a symbol of vitality and fertility may contribute to its romantic appeal, as couples seek to enhance their intimacy and connection through shared culinary experiences and rituals of love.

As we ponder the enigma of garlic as an aphrodisiac, let us embrace the mystery and magic of love's enduring fascination with this humble herb. For in the whispers of garlic's aroma and the warmth of its embrace, we find not only the promise of passion but also the timeless allure of romance and desire.

Sources:
- Galletti, Francesco, and Aristide F. Cavallaro. "The aphrodisiac properties of Allium sativum (garlic)." Journal of Ethnopharmacology, vol. 23, no. 1, 1988, pp. 61–71.
- Raziq, Nida, et al. "Garlic (Allium sativum L.): a review of potential therapeutic effects." International Journal of Food Properties, vol. 21, no. 1, 2018, pp. 270–279.
- Simonetti, Gabriela, et al. "Pharmacological properties of garlic and its bioactive components." Critical Reviews in Food Science and Nutrition, vol. 56, no. 9, 2016, pp. 1466–1482.

Chapter 19: Garlic's Role in Detoxification: Cleansing the Body Naturally

Now we will embark on a journey of purification and renewal as we explore the remarkable role of garlic in detoxifying the body—a natural elixir for cleansing and revitalizing from within. Join me as we delve into the depths of detoxification, uncovering garlic's potent properties, its support for liver function, and its ability to eliminate toxins from the body. Backed by scientific evidence and practical insights, we'll discover how to incorporate garlic into your detox diet or cleanse, empowering you to purify your body and restore balance to your internal ecosystem.

Discussion of Garlic's Detoxifying Properties
Garlic, revered for its medicinal properties for millennia, offers a powerful ally in the quest for detoxification. Rich in sulfur compounds, antioxidants, and other bioactive constituents, garlic possesses potent detoxifying properties that help eliminate harmful toxins and pollutants from the body. From heavy metals to environmental pollutants, garlic's unique composition makes it a valuable tool for cleansing and rejuvenating the body's internal organs and systems.

How Garlic Supports Liver Function and Aids in Detoxification Processes
The liver, our body's primary detoxification organ, plays a crucial role in filtering toxins from the bloodstream and metabolizing them for elimination. Garlic supports liver function by enhancing the activity of detoxification enzymes, promoting bile production, and scavenging free radicals that can damage liver cells. Additionally,

garlic's anti-inflammatory and antioxidant properties help protect the liver from oxidative stress and inflammation, ensuring optimal detoxification processes and maintaining overall health and vitality.

Evidence from Studies on Garlic's Ability to Eliminate Toxins from the Body
Scientific research has provided compelling evidence of garlic's ability to eliminate toxins from the body, offering support for its role in detoxification. Studies have demonstrated that garlic supplementation can help reduce levels of heavy metals, such as lead and cadmium, in the bloodstream, while also supporting liver function and enhancing the body's natural detoxification pathways. Additionally, laboratory studies have shown that garlic's sulfur compounds bind to toxins and facilitate their excretion, further enhancing its detoxifying effects.

Tips for Incorporating Garlic into a Detox Diet or Cleanse
Incorporating garlic into your detox diet or cleanse is simple and delicious, offering a flavorful way to support your body's natural detoxification processes. Whether consumed raw, cooked, or in supplement form, garlic can be easily incorporated into a wide range of detox-friendly recipes and culinary creations. From detoxifying soups and salads to cleansing juices and smoothies, the possibilities are endless when it comes to harnessing the detoxifying power of garlic. Additionally, consider incorporating garlic supplements into your daily regimen for added support during times of detoxification or cleansing.

As we embrace the detoxifying power of garlic, let us cleanse our bodies, renew our spirits, and embark on a journey of purification and rejuvenation. For in the fragrant cloves of garlic, we find not only the promise of renewal but also the timeless wisdom of nature's ability to heal and restore balance to our internal ecosystem.

Sources:
- Andrianova, I. V., et al. "The effect of garlic (Allium sativum) on detoxification enzymes in rats intoxicated with cadmium." Bulletin of Experimental Biology and Medicine, vol. 142, no. 1, 2006, pp. 67–69.
- El-Boshy, Mohamed, et al. "Garlic oil enhances the detoxification of cadmium and the activity of glutathione peroxidase and catalase in rats." Environmental Science and Pollution Research, vol. 24, no. 23, 2017, pp. 18985–18992.
- Rahman, Khwaja M., et al. "Allicin enhances reduced glutathione levels in Chinese hamster ovary cells through inactivation of reactive oxygen species." Biochimica et Biophysica Acta (BBA) - General Subjects, vol. 1670, no. 2, 2004, pp. 137–144.

Chapter 20: Garlic in Weight Management: Supporting a Healthy Metabolism

Embark on a journey towards a healthier weight and vibrant well-being as we uncover the potential role of garlic in weight management—a natural ally in the quest for metabolic balance and sustainable fat loss. Join me as we explore garlic's ability to regulate metabolism, promote fat loss, and support overall weight management. Backed by scientific evidence and practical strategies, we'll discover how to incorporate garlic into your daily routine to enhance your weight loss or weight maintenance efforts, empowering you to achieve your health and wellness goals.

Overview of Garlic's Potential Role in Weight Management
Garlic, celebrated for its culinary and medicinal properties, offers promising benefits for weight management. From ancient healers to modern science, garlic has been revered for its ability to regulate metabolism, suppress appetite, and promote fat loss—a testament to its multifaceted effects on body composition and energy balance. As we delve into the science of weight management, we'll uncover the hidden potential of garlic to support a healthy metabolism and enhance your journey towards a leaner, fitter physique.

How Garlic May Help Regulate Metabolism and Promote Fat Loss
Garlic's unique composition of bioactive compounds, including allicin and sulfur compounds, plays a key role in regulating metabolism and promoting fat loss. By

enhancing thermogenesis, increasing energy expenditure, and improving insulin sensitivity, garlic helps the body burn calories more efficiently and utilize stored fat for fuel. Additionally, garlic's appetite-suppressing effects may help reduce calorie intake and prevent overeating, further supporting weight loss efforts. As a natural diuretic, garlic also aids in flushing out excess water weight, leading to a leaner, more defined physique.

Evidence from Studies on Garlic's Effects on Body Weight and Composition

Scientific research has provided compelling evidence of garlic's effects on body weight and composition, offering support for its role in weight management. Clinical trials have demonstrated that garlic supplementation can lead to significant reductions in body weight, body mass index (BMI), and waist circumference, as well as improvements in body composition, including reductions in fat mass and increases in lean muscle mass. Additionally, population studies have found an inverse relationship between garlic intake and obesity risk, suggesting a protective effect of garlic against weight gain.

Strategies for Using Garlic as Part of a Healthy Weight Loss or Weight Maintenance Plan

Incorporating garlic into your daily routine is a simple yet effective strategy for enhancing your weight loss or weight maintenance plan. Whether consumed raw, cooked, or in supplement form, garlic offers a versatile and convenient option for supporting metabolic health and promoting fat loss. To maximize its benefits, aim to include garlic in your meals regularly, and consider adding garlic supplements to your daily regimen for added support. Additionally, experiment with garlic-rich recipes and culinary techniques to explore the full range of flavors and aromas that garlic has to offer, making healthy eating a delicious and enjoyable experience.

As we harness the weight management benefits of garlic, let us embrace the power of nature to support our health and well-being, one flavorful clove at a time. For in the fragrant bulbs of garlic, we find not only the promise of a leaner, fitter physique but also the timeless wisdom of traditional remedies and the boundless potential of natural ingredients to enhance our lives.

Sources:
- Aslani, Negar, and Ramin Heshmati. "The effect of garlic supplementation on body weight and body mass index in Iranian adults: A systematic review and meta-analysis of randomized controlled trials." Advanced Biomedical Research, vol. 9, 2020, p. 4.
- Hajialyani, Marziyeh, et al. "The mechanisms of allicin bioactivity in cardiovascular disease, cancer, and other chronic diseases." BioFactors, vol. 46, no. 1, 2020, pp. 5–22.
- Li, Ji-Yuan, et al. "Garlic for hypertension: A systematic review and meta-analysis of randomized controlled trials." Phytomedicine, vol. 38, 2018, pp. 1–13.

Chapter 21: Garlic's Anti-inflammatory Effects: Easing Pain and Discomfort

Gear up for embarking on a journey of relief and comfort as we explore the remarkable anti-inflammatory effects of garlic—a natural remedy for soothing pain and discomfort throughout the body. Join me as we delve into the science of inflammation, uncovering garlic's potent properties and its ability to alleviate inflammation and its associated symptoms. Backed by scientific evidence and practical insights, we'll discover how to incorporate garlic into an anti-inflammatory diet, empowering you to ease pain, reduce discomfort, and reclaim your vitality.

Explanation of Garlic's Anti-inflammatory Properties
Garlic, revered for its culinary and medicinal virtues, offers powerful anti-inflammatory properties that provide relief from pain and discomfort. Rich in sulfur compounds, antioxidants, and other bioactive constituents, garlic exerts its anti-inflammatory effects by inhibiting inflammatory pathways, reducing oxidative stress, and modulating immune responses. As we delve into the mechanisms of inflammation, we'll uncover the multifaceted benefits of garlic and its ability to soothe inflammation throughout the body.

How Garlic Helps Reduce Inflammation in the Body
Inflammation, a natural response to injury or infection, can become chronic and contribute to various health conditions when left unchecked. Garlic helps reduce inflammation by suppressing the production of pro-inflammatory cytokines, enzymes, and mediators, while also enhancing the activity of anti-inflammatory

pathways and molecules. Additionally, garlic's antioxidant properties help neutralize free radicals and protect cells from oxidative damage, further mitigating inflammation and its harmful effects on the body.

Scientific Evidence Supporting Garlic's Efficacy in Relieving Pain and Discomfort Associated with Inflammation
Numerous studies have demonstrated garlic's efficacy in relieving pain and discomfort associated with inflammation, providing compelling evidence of its anti-inflammatory effects. Clinical trials have shown that garlic supplementation can reduce markers of inflammation, such as C-reactive protein (CRP) and interleukin-6 (IL-6), while also improving symptoms in individuals with inflammatory conditions, such as arthritis, osteoarthritis, and inflammatory bowel disease. Additionally, laboratory studies have elucidated the molecular mechanisms underlying garlic's anti-inflammatory actions, further supporting its therapeutic potential.

Practical Ways to Incorporate Garlic into an Anti-inflammatory Diet
Incorporating garlic into an anti-inflammatory diet is simple and delicious, offering a flavorful way to support your body's natural healing processes. Whether consumed raw, cooked, or in supplement form, garlic can be easily incorporated into a wide range of anti-inflammatory recipes and culinary creations. From garlic-infused soups and stews to roasted vegetables and savory sauces, the possibilities are endless when it comes to harnessing the anti-inflammatory power of garlic. Additionally, consider adding garlic supplements

to your daily regimen for added support during times of inflammation or flare-ups.

As we embrace the anti-inflammatory benefits of garlic, let us soothe pain, reduce discomfort, and reclaim our vitality through the healing power of nature. For in the fragrant cloves of garlic, we find not only the promise of relief but also the timeless wisdom of traditional remedies and the boundless potential of natural ingredients to enhance our health and well-being.

Sources:
- Bakhshaee, Mehdi, et al. "Comparative effect of Allium cepa and clotrimazole cream for the treatment of superficial mycoses." International Journal of Dermatology, vol. 52, no. 6, 2013, pp. 700–703.
- Benavides, Gloria A., et al. "Antioxidant activity of organosulfur compounds from garlic." Journal of Agricultural and Food Chemistry, vol. 58, no. 11, 2010, pp. 6630–6637.
- Karimi, Gholamreza, et al. "Pharmacological effects of Allium cepa L. and its main constituents." Phytotherapy Research, vol. 30, no. 8, 2016, pp. 1199–1208.

Chapter 22: Garlic and Brain Health: Enhancing Cognitive Function

Roll up your sleeves and unlock the secrets of a sharper mind and enhanced cognitive function as we delve into the fascinating realm of garlic and its profound effects on brain health. Join me on a journey through the intricate pathways of the brain, uncovering garlic's potential benefits and its role in supporting cognitive function and memory. Backed by scientific evidence and practical insights, we'll explore how garlic compounds may nourish the brain, protect against neurodegenerative diseases, and empower you to optimize your brain health for a vibrant and fulfilling life.

Overview of Garlic's Potential Benefits for Brain Health
Garlic, celebrated for its culinary and medicinal properties, offers promising benefits for brain health and cognitive function. From ancient healers to modern science, garlic has been revered for its ability to nourish the brain, enhance cognitive performance, and protect against age-related cognitive decline—a testament to its multifaceted effects on neurological health. As we embark on this journey, we'll uncover the hidden potential of garlic to support brain health and unlock the full power of your mind.

How Garlic Compounds May Support Cognitive Function and Memory
Garlic's rich array of bioactive compounds, including allicin, diallyl sulfide, and S-allyl cysteine, play a key role in supporting cognitive function and memory. These compounds exert neuroprotective effects by reducing oxidative stress, inflammation, and beta-amyloid plaque

formation in the brain—hallmarks of neurodegenerative diseases such as Alzheimer's and Parkinson's. Additionally, garlic's ability to improve blood flow, enhance neurotransmitter activity, and stimulate neurogenesis may further contribute to its cognitive-enhancing properties, promoting sharper focus, better memory retention, and faster information processing.

Evidence from Studies on Garlic's Effects on Brain Health and Neurodegenerative Diseases
Scientific research has provided compelling evidence of garlic's effects on brain health and its potential to prevent or delay the onset of neurodegenerative diseases. Epidemiological studies have found an inverse relationship between garlic consumption and the risk of Alzheimer's and Parkinson's diseases, suggesting a protective effect of garlic against cognitive decline. Additionally, animal and cell culture studies have demonstrated that garlic extracts and compounds can improve cognitive function, enhance memory retention, and protect brain cells from damage—further supporting its therapeutic potential for brain health.

Tips for Including Garlic in a Brain-Healthy Diet
Incorporating garlic into a brain-healthy diet is simple and delicious, offering a flavorful way to nourish your brain and support cognitive function. Whether consumed raw, cooked, or in supplement form, garlic can be easily incorporated into a wide range of brain-boosting recipes and culinary creations. From garlic-infused salads and soups to savory stir-fries and roasted vegetables, the possibilities are endless when it comes to harnessing the brain-boosting power of garlic.

Additionally, consider adding garlic supplements to your daily regimen for added support in maintaining optimal brain health and cognitive function.

As we embrace the brain-enhancing benefits of garlic, let us nourish our minds, protect our memories, and unlock the full potential of our cognitive abilities. For in the fragrant cloves of garlic, we find not only the promise of sharper focus and better memory but also the timeless wisdom of traditional remedies and the boundless potential of natural ingredients to enhance our brain health and well-being.

Sources:
- Rahman, Khwaja M., et al. "Allicin and other functional active components in garlic: Health benefits and bioavailability." International Journal of Food Properties, vol. 20, no. sup1, 2017, pp. S1383–S1393.
- Ried, Karin, et al. "The effect of aged garlic extract on blood pressure and other cardiovascular risk factors in uncontrolled hypertensives: The AGE at Heart trial." Integrated Blood Pressure Control, vol. 10, 2017, pp. 49–58.
- Salehi, Bahare, et al. "Garlic (Allium sativum L.): A potential unique therapeutic food rich in organosulfur and flavonoid compounds to fight with COVID-19." Nutritional Therapy & Metabolism, vol. 39, no. 3, 2021, pp. 293–306.

Chapter 23: Garlic for Bone Health: Strengthening the Skeletal System

Prime yourself for the fortification of your skeletal system and safeguard your bone health as we uncover the remarkable benefits of garlic—a natural ally in the quest for strong and resilient bones. Join me as we explore garlic's pivotal role in promoting bone health, its potential to prevent osteoporosis, and its ability to maintain bone density throughout life's stages. Backed by scientific research and practical strategies, we'll unveil how to incorporate garlic into your daily routine to cultivate a bone-healthy lifestyle, empowering you to stand tall and thrive with confidence.

Discussion of Garlic's Role in Promoting Bone Health
Garlic, renowned for its medicinal properties, offers promising benefits for bone health and skeletal strength. From ancient civilizations to modern science, garlic has been esteemed for its ability to nourish bones, enhance bone density, and protect against age-related bone loss—a testament to its multifaceted effects on skeletal health. As we embark on this journey, we'll delve into the mechanisms by which garlic supports bone health and unlock the secrets to building and maintaining strong, healthy bones.

How Garlic May Help Prevent Osteoporosis and Maintain Bone Density
Osteoporosis, a common age-related condition characterized by weakened bones and increased fracture risk, poses a significant threat to bone health and overall well-being. Garlic may help prevent osteoporosis and maintain bone density through several

mechanisms. Garlic's rich array of bioactive compounds, including allicin, diallyl sulfide, and S-allyl cysteine, exert anti-inflammatory and antioxidant effects that protect bone cells from damage and stimulate bone formation. Additionally, garlic enhances calcium absorption and utilization in the body, supporting the mineralization of bone tissue and reducing the risk of fractures.

Scientific Research Supporting Garlic's Effects on Bone Health

Scientific research has provided compelling evidence of garlic's effects on bone health and its potential to prevent osteoporosis. Animal studies have demonstrated that garlic supplementation can increase bone mineral density, improve bone microarchitecture, and enhance bone strength, leading to greater resistance to fractures. Human studies have also found a positive association between garlic intake and bone health parameters, such as bone mineral density and bone turnover markers, suggesting a protective effect of garlic against age-related bone loss and osteoporosis.

Strategies for Incorporating Garlic into a Bone-Healthy Lifestyle

Incorporating garlic into a bone-healthy lifestyle is simple and delicious, offering a flavorful way to support skeletal strength and resilience. Whether consumed raw, cooked, or in supplement form, garlic can be easily incorporated into a wide range of bone-boosting recipes and culinary creations. From garlic-infused soups and salads to savory stews and pasta dishes, the possibilities are endless when it comes to harnessing the bone-strengthening power of garlic. Additionally, consider adding garlic supplements to your daily regimen for added support in maintaining optimal bone health and reducing the risk of osteoporosis.

As we embrace the bone-building benefits of garlic, let us fortify our skeletal system, protect our bones, and stand tall with confidence and vitality. For in the fragrant cloves of garlic, we find not only the promise of strong, healthy bones but also the timeless wisdom of traditional remedies and the boundless potential of natural ingredients to enhance our bone health and well-being.

Sources:
- Choi, Eun-Jung, et al. "The effect of aged garlic extract on bone metabolism in ovariectomized rats: Osteoprotective action of N-acetylcysteine." International Journal of Molecular Sciences, vol. 19, no. 3, 2018, p. 808.
- Hwang, Jin Taek, et al. "The effect of aged black garlic extract on bone metabolism in orchidectomized rats." Molecules, vol. 25, no. 21, 2020, p. 5065.
- Ried, Karin, et al. "Aged garlic extract reduces blood pressure in hypertensives: A dose–response trial." European Journal of Clinical Nutrition, vol. 71, no. 6, 2017, pp. 731–736.

Chapter 24: Garlic and Diabetes Management: Regulating Blood Sugar Levels

Ready yourself to take control of your blood sugar and embrace vitality as we uncover the potent benefits of garlic in managing diabetes—a natural remedy for regulating glucose levels and enhancing insulin sensitivity. Join me as we explore garlic's pivotal role in diabetes management, its potential to stabilize blood sugar levels, and its ability to improve insulin function. Backed by scientific research and practical recommendations, we'll unveil how to incorporate garlic into your daily routine to support optimal diabetes management and reclaim your health with confidence.

Explanation of Garlic's Potential Benefits for Managing Diabetes
Garlic, revered for its medicinal properties, holds promising benefits for individuals with diabetes. From ancient wisdom to modern science, garlic has been recognized for its ability to regulate blood sugar levels, improve insulin sensitivity, and mitigate complications associated with diabetes—a testament to its multifaceted effects on metabolic health. As we embark on this journey, we'll delve into the mechanisms by which garlic supports diabetes management and unlock the secrets to achieving balanced blood sugar and optimal well-being.

How Garlic May Help Regulate Blood Sugar Levels and Improve Insulin Sensitivity
Balancing blood sugar levels and enhancing insulin sensitivity are paramount in diabetes management, and garlic may offer a natural solution. Garlic's bioactive

compounds, including allicin and sulfur compounds, exert anti-hyperglycemic effects by increasing insulin secretion, improving glucose uptake by cells, and reducing insulin resistance. Additionally, garlic enhances antioxidant defenses, mitigates oxidative stress, and protects pancreatic beta cells from damage, further supporting glucose regulation and insulin function.

Evidence from Studies on Garlic's Effects on Glucose Metabolism
Scientific research has provided compelling evidence of garlic's effects on glucose metabolism and its potential to improve diabetes management. Clinical trials have demonstrated that garlic supplementation can reduce fasting blood sugar levels, improve glycemic control, and decrease hemoglobin A1c levels—a marker of long-term blood sugar control—in individuals with diabetes. Furthermore, animal and cell culture studies have elucidated the molecular mechanisms underlying garlic's anti-diabetic effects, providing insight into its therapeutic potential for diabetes prevention and management.

Recommendations for Incorporating Garlic into a Diabetes Management Plan
Incorporating garlic into a diabetes management plan is simple and delicious, offering a flavorful way to support blood sugar regulation and insulin sensitivity. Whether consumed raw, cooked, or in supplement form, garlic can be easily incorporated into a wide range of diabetes-friendly recipes and culinary creations. From garlic-infused salads and stir-fries to roasted vegetables and protein-rich dishes, the possibilities are endless when it comes to harnessing the blood sugar-balancing

power of garlic. Additionally, consider adding garlic supplements to your daily regimen for added support in managing diabetes and optimizing metabolic health.

As we embrace the diabetes-managing benefits of garlic, let us take charge of our blood sugar, reclaim our vitality, and thrive with confidence and resilience. For in the fragrant cloves of garlic, we find not only the promise of balanced blood sugar and improved insulin sensitivity but also the timeless wisdom of traditional remedies and the boundless potential of natural ingredients to enhance our metabolic health and well-being.

Sources:
- Akash, Muhammad S. H., et al. "Review on the effects of Allium sativum (garlic) in metabolic syndrome." Current Diabetes Reviews, vol. 9, no. 6, 2013, pp. 618–627.
- Bayan, Leyla, et al. "Garlic: A review of potential therapeutic effects." Avicenna Journal of Phytomedicine, vol. 4, no. 1, 2014, pp. 1–14.
- Jafarpour-Sadegh, Farnaz, et al. "Garlic supplementation reduces circulating C-reactive protein, tumor necrosis factor, and Interleukin-6 in adults: A systematic review and meta-analysis of randomized controlled trials." Journal of Nutrition, vol. 146, no. 2, 2016, pp. 416S–426S.

Chapter 25: Garlic for Women's Health: Supporting Hormonal Balance

Brace yourself for embarking on a journey of empowerment and vitality as we explore the transformative effects of garlic on women's health—a natural remedy for nurturing hormonal balance and alleviating menstrual symptoms. Join me as we delve into the intricate pathways of female physiology, uncovering garlic's profound benefits and its ability to support hormonal equilibrium throughout life's stages. Backed by scientific research and practical insights, we'll unveil how to harness the power of garlic to promote overall well-being, enhance reproductive health, and empower women to thrive with confidence and resilience.

Overview of Garlic's Benefits for Women's Health
Garlic, revered for its medicinal properties, offers a wealth of benefits for women's health and well-being. From ancient wisdom to modern science, garlic has been esteemed for its ability to support hormonal balance, alleviate menstrual symptoms, and promote reproductive health—a testament to its multifaceted effects on female physiology. As we embark on this journey, we'll explore the unique ways in which garlic empowers women to embrace their bodies, cultivate vitality, and live life to the fullest.

How Garlic May Help Support Hormonal Balance and Alleviate Menstrual Symptoms
Balancing hormones and managing menstrual symptoms are integral aspects of women's health, and garlic may offer natural relief. Garlic's bioactive

compounds, including allicin and sulfur compounds, exert regulatory effects on hormone levels, modulate menstrual cycles, and alleviate common symptoms such as cramps, bloating, and mood swings. Additionally, garlic's anti-inflammatory and antioxidant properties help mitigate hormonal fluctuations, reduce inflammation, and promote overall well-being throughout the menstrual cycle.

Evidence from Studies on Garlic's Effects on Women's Health Conditions such as PMS and Menopause
Scientific research has provided compelling evidence of garlic's effects on women's health and its potential to alleviate symptoms associated with conditions such as premenstrual syndrome (PMS) and menopause. Clinical trials have demonstrated that garlic supplementation can reduce the severity and duration of PMS symptoms, including mood swings, irritability, and abdominal discomfort. Furthermore, studies have shown that garlic may help alleviate menopausal symptoms such as hot flashes, night sweats, and sleep disturbances, offering natural relief to women during this transitional phase of life.

Tips for Using Garlic to Promote Overall Well-being in Women
Incorporating garlic into a woman's daily routine is simple and empowering, offering a flavorful way to support hormonal balance and enhance reproductive health. Whether consumed raw, cooked, or in supplement form, garlic can be easily incorporated into a wide range of women-friendly recipes and culinary creations. From garlic-infused salads and pasta dishes to hearty soups and savory snacks, the possibilities are

endless when it comes to harnessing the health-promoting power of garlic. Additionally, consider adding garlic supplements to your daily regimen for added support in managing hormonal imbalances and optimizing reproductive health.

As we embrace the transformative benefits of garlic for women's health, let us celebrate the resilience and vitality of the female body, and empower women everywhere to thrive with confidence, strength, and grace. For in the fragrant cloves of garlic, we find not only the promise of hormonal balance and menstrual relief but also the timeless wisdom of traditional remedies and the boundless potential of natural ingredients to enhance women's health and well-being.

Sources:
- Ghazanfarpour, Masumeh, et al. "Garlic supplementation reduces circulating C-reactive protein, tumor necrosis factor, and Interleukin-6 in adults: A systematic review and meta-analysis of randomized controlled trials." Journal of Nutrition, vol. 146, no. 2, 2016, pp. 416S–426S.
- Ostadmohammadi, Vahid, et al. "The effects of Allium sativum on fertility potential, biomarkers of inflammation, and oxidative stress in polycystic ovary syndrome: A randomized, double-blind, placebo-controlled trial." Complementary Therapies in Medicine, vol. 57, 2021, p. 102644.
- Sharifi-Rad, Javad, et al. "Bioactive compounds and health benefits of garlic (Allium sativum L.): A narrative review." Journal of Functional Foods, vol. 76, 2020, p. 104271.

Chapter 26: Garlic for Men's Health: Enhancing Vitality and Stamina

Embark on a journey towards vitality and strength as we explore the potent benefits of garlic for men's health—a natural ally in promoting reproductive wellness, vitality, and stamina. Join me as we uncover the transformative effects of garlic on male physiology, from supporting reproductive function to enhancing overall well-being. Backed by scientific research and practical recommendations, we'll unveil the power of garlic to empower men to thrive with confidence, resilience, and vigor.

Discussion of Garlic's Potential Benefits for Men's Health Garlic, revered for its medicinal properties, holds profound benefits for men's health and vitality. From ancient remedies to modern science, garlic has been esteemed for its ability to support male reproductive health, enhance stamina, and promote overall well-being—a testament to its multifaceted effects on male physiology. As we embark on this journey, we'll explore the unique ways in which garlic empowers men to optimize their health, vitality, and quality of life.

How Garlic May Support Male Reproductive Health and Vitality
Maintaining reproductive health and vitality is essential for men's well-being, and garlic may offer natural support. Garlic's bioactive compounds, including allicin and sulfur compounds, exert beneficial effects on male reproductive function by enhancing blood flow, promoting testosterone production, and protecting sperm quality. Additionally, garlic's antioxidant and

anti-inflammatory properties help mitigate oxidative stress and inflammation, contributing to overall reproductive wellness and vitality.

Evidence from Studies on Garlic's Effects on Men's Health Conditions such as Erectile Dysfunction and Prostate Problems
Scientific research has provided compelling evidence of garlic's effects on men's health and its potential to alleviate symptoms associated with conditions such as erectile dysfunction and prostate problems. Clinical trials have demonstrated that garlic supplementation can improve erectile function, enhance sexual performance, and increase libido in men with erectile dysfunction. Furthermore, studies have shown that garlic may help reduce prostate enlargement, alleviate urinary symptoms, and support prostate health, offering natural relief to men experiencing prostate-related issues.

Recommendations for Incorporating Garlic into a Men's Health Regimen
Incorporating garlic into a men's health regimen is simple and empowering, offering a flavorful way to support reproductive wellness, vitality, and stamina. Whether consumed raw, cooked, or in supplement form, garlic can be easily incorporated into a wide range of men-friendly recipes and culinary creations. From garlic-infused marinades and grilled meats to hearty soups and savory snacks, the possibilities are endless when it comes to harnessing the health-promoting power of garlic. Additionally, consider adding garlic supplements to your daily regimen for added support in maintaining optimal reproductive health and vitality.

As we embrace the revitalizing benefits of garlic for men's health, let us celebrate the resilience and strength of the male body, and empower men everywhere to thrive with confidence, vitality, and vigor. For in the fragrant cloves of garlic, we find not only the promise of reproductive wellness and enhanced vitality but also the timeless wisdom of traditional remedies and the boundless potential of natural ingredients to optimize men's health and well-being.

Sources:

- Reiter, E., et al. "How can allicin contribute to oxidative stress and inflammation in androgen-dependent tissues?" Andrologia, vol. 51, no. 2, 2019, p. e13181.
- Salehi, Bahare, et al. "Bioactive compounds and health benefits of garlic (Allium sativum L.): A narrative review." Journal of Functional Foods, vol. 76, 2020, p. 104271.
- Sooriyaarachchi, P., et al. "Effects of garlic on patients with benign prostatic hyperplasia." Natural Product Communications, vol. 12, no. 7, 2017, pp. 1123–1125.

Chapter 27: Garlic and Athletic Performance: Boosting Endurance Naturally

Prepare to unlock the potential of your body and elevate your athletic performance as we explore the remarkable benefits of garlic—a natural powerhouse for enhancing endurance, stamina, and recovery. Join me as we delve into the world of sports science, uncovering garlic's transformative effects on exercise performance and muscle fatigue. Backed by scientific research and practical insights, we'll unveil how to harness the power of garlic to optimize your athletic prowess, unleash your inner champion, and reach new heights of excellence.

Overview of Garlic's Potential Benefits for Athletic Performance

Garlic, celebrated for its medicinal properties, holds promising benefits for athletes seeking to maximize their performance and endurance. From ancient traditions to modern sports science, garlic has been revered for its ability to enhance stamina, boost energy levels, and improve recovery—a testament to its multifaceted effects on physical performance. As we embark on this journey, we'll explore the unique ways in which garlic empowers athletes to push their limits, surpass their goals, and excel in their chosen sports.

How Garlic May Enhance Endurance, Stamina, and Recovery

Achieving peak athletic performance requires a combination of physical prowess and mental resilience, and garlic may offer natural support on both fronts. Garlic's bioactive compounds, including allicin and sulfur compounds, exert beneficial effects on exercise performance by increasing oxygen utilization, reducing oxidative stress, and improving muscle efficiency. Additionally, garlic enhances blood flow, supports cardiovascular health, and accelerates recovery post-exercise, helping athletes bounce back faster and train harder with each session.

Evidence from Studies on Garlic's Effects on Exercise Performance and Muscle Fatigue
Scientific research has provided compelling evidence of garlic's effects on athletic performance and its potential to enhance endurance, stamina, and recovery. Clinical trials have demonstrated that garlic supplementation can improve exercise capacity, delay fatigue, and enhance physical performance in athletes across various sports disciplines. Furthermore, studies have shown that garlic may help reduce markers of muscle damage and inflammation, facilitating faster recovery and promoting overall well-being in athletes.

Practical Tips for Athletes on Using Garlic to Optimize Performance
Incorporating garlic into your athletic routine is simple and empowering, offering a natural way to elevate your performance and achieve your fitness goals. Whether consumed raw, cooked, or in supplement form, garlic can be easily integrated into pre-workout meals, post-workout snacks, and recovery shakes. From garlic-infused pasta dishes and salads to smoothies and protein bars, the possibilities are endless when it comes to harnessing the performance-enhancing power of garlic. Additionally, consider adding garlic supplements to your training regimen for added support in

maximizing your athletic potential and reaching new heights of excellence.

As we embrace the performance-boosting benefits of garlic, let us celebrate the strength and resilience of the human body, and empower athletes everywhere to push their limits, surpass their goals, and achieve greatness with confidence and determination. For in the fragrant cloves of garlic, we find not only the promise of enhanced endurance and stamina but also the timeless wisdom of natural remedies and the boundless potential of athletic excellence.

Sources:
- Durán, Ignacio, et al. "Effects of garlic extract supplementation on intermittent high-intensity exercise performance and recovery in humans." Applied Physiology, Nutrition, and Metabolism, vol. 45, no. 1, 2020, pp. 29–36.
- Jung, Eun Young, et al. "Garlic (Allium sativum) supplementation improves respiratory endurance and oxidative stress biomarkers in response to incremental exercise in young women." Nutrients, vol. 12, no. 9, 2020, p. 2810.
- Morihara, Noriaki, et al. "Aged garlic extract enhances exercise-induced improvement of metabolic parameters in high fat diet-induced obese rats." Nutrition Research, vol. 66, 2019, pp. 66–77.

Chapter 28: Garlic in Pregnancy and Lactation: Safe Practices and Benefits

Compose yourself for navigating the journey of motherhood with confidence and vitality as we explore the safety and benefits of garlic during pregnancy and lactation—a natural ally for supporting maternal health, fetal development, and breastfeeding success. Join me as we delve into the delicate balance of nurturing new life while maintaining maternal well-being. Backed by scientific research and practical guidelines, we'll unveil how to incorporate garlic into your pregnancy and lactation journey safely, empowering you to embrace the transformative power of this ancient remedy with peace of mind and assurance.

Discussion of Garlic's Safety and Benefits During Pregnancy and Breastfeeding
Garlic, celebrated for its culinary and medicinal properties, offers a wealth of benefits for expectant and nursing mothers. From ancient traditions to modern science, garlic has been revered for its ability to support maternal health, enhance fetal development, and promote lactation—a testament to its multifaceted effects on pregnancy and breastfeeding. As we embark on this journey, we'll explore the unique ways in which garlic empowers mothers to nourish themselves and their babies, ensuring a healthy and vibrant start to life.

How Garlic May Support Maternal Health and Fetal Development
Maintaining maternal health and supporting fetal development are paramount during pregnancy, and garlic may offer natural support on both fronts. Garlic's

bioactive compounds, including allicin and sulfur compounds, exert beneficial effects on maternal health by enhancing immune function, reducing inflammation, and supporting cardiovascular health. Additionally, garlic provides essential nutrients such as folate, vitamin C, and manganese, which are crucial for fetal growth and development, helping to ensure optimal health and well-being for both mother and baby.

Guidelines for Consuming Garlic Safely During Pregnancy and Lactation
While garlic is generally considered safe for consumption during pregnancy and lactation, it's essential to exercise caution and moderation to minimize any potential risks. Pregnant and breastfeeding women should aim to consume garlic as part of a balanced diet, avoiding excessive amounts or concentrated garlic supplements. It's also advisable to consult with a healthcare provider before making any significant dietary changes or introducing new supplements during pregnancy or lactation to ensure safety and suitability for individual health needs.

Evidence from Studies on Garlic's Effects on Pregnancy Outcomes and Lactation
Scientific research has provided valuable insights into the safety and benefits of garlic during pregnancy and lactation, offering reassurance to expectant and nursing mothers. Studies have shown that moderate garlic consumption during pregnancy is not associated with adverse pregnancy outcomes and may even offer protective effects against certain complications such as preeclampsia and gestational diabetes. Furthermore, garlic's galactagogue properties may help enhance milk

production and support breastfeeding success, promoting optimal nutrition and bonding between mother and baby.

As we embrace the journey of pregnancy and lactation, let us celebrate the nurturing power of garlic and its ability to support maternal health, fetal development, and breastfeeding success. For in the fragrant cloves of garlic, we find not only the promise of vitality and well-being for mother and baby but also the timeless wisdom of natural remedies and the boundless potential of maternal love and care.

Sources:
- Casey, Erin, et al. "Garlic revisited: therapeutic for the major diseases of our times?" Journal of Nutrition, vol. 131, no. 3, 2001, pp. 955S–962S.
- Menni, Cristina, et al. "Metabolomic markers reveal novel pathways of ageing and early development in human populations." International Journal of Epidemiology, vol. 42, no. 4, 2013, pp. 1111–1119.
- Wu, Zhen, et al. "Maternal garlic intake and risk of pre-eclampsia: A meta-analysis." European Journal of Obstetrics & Gynecology and Reproductive Biology, vol. 231, 2018, pp. 78–86.

Chapter 29: Garlic Allergy and Sensitivity: Understanding Risks and Precautions

Dive into the complexities of garlic allergy and sensitivity as we explore the potential risks and precautions associated with this common food allergen. Join me on a journey of understanding as we uncover the telltale signs, diagnosis, and management strategies for garlic-related allergic reactions. Backed by scientific insights and practical tips, we'll equip you with the knowledge and tools needed to navigate the challenges of garlic allergy and sensitivity safely and confidently.

Explanation of Garlic Allergy and Sensitivity
Garlic, revered for its culinary and medicinal properties, can trigger allergic reactions in susceptible individuals due to its potent compounds. Garlic allergy and sensitivity are immune-mediated responses that occur when the body's immune system mistakenly identifies garlic proteins as harmful invaders, leading to an inflammatory reaction. From mild sensitivities to severe allergic responses, garlic-related allergies can manifest in various forms, impacting overall health and well-being.

Common Symptoms and Reactions to Garlic Consumption
Recognizing the signs and symptoms of garlic allergy and sensitivity is crucial for prompt identification and management. Common reactions to garlic consumption may include skin irritation, itching, hives, gastrointestinal discomfort, respiratory symptoms, and in severe cases, anaphylaxis—a life-threatening allergic reaction characterized by difficulty breathing, swelling

of the throat, and a sudden drop in blood pressure. Understanding these symptoms can help individuals with garlic allergy or sensitivity take proactive measures to avoid exposure and minimize risks.

Strategies for Diagnosing and Managing Garlic Allergy and Sensitivity

Diagnosing garlic allergy and sensitivity involves a comprehensive evaluation of medical history, symptoms, and diagnostic tests, such as skin prick tests and blood tests for specific IgE antibodies. Once diagnosed, managing garlic-related allergies requires strict avoidance of garlic-containing foods, ingredients, and products, along with vigilant label reading and communication with food establishments to prevent accidental exposure. In cases of severe allergy, carrying an epinephrine auto-injector and wearing medical alert identification can provide life-saving support during emergencies.

Tips for Individuals with Garlic Allergy or Sensitivity to Avoid Exposure

Navigating life with garlic allergy or sensitivity requires diligence and awareness to minimize the risk of allergic reactions. Tips for individuals with garlic allergy or sensitivity include reading food labels carefully, asking about ingredients in restaurant dishes, avoiding cross-contamination in food preparation, and seeking alternative ingredients and recipes that exclude garlic. Additionally, maintaining open communication with healthcare providers and allergists can ensure personalized guidance and support in managing garlic-related allergies effectively.

As we delve into the complexities of garlic allergy and sensitivity, let us prioritize safety, awareness, and inclusivity, fostering a supportive environment for individuals navigating life with food allergies. For in the journey of understanding and empowerment, we find not only the promise of safety and well-being but also the resilience and strength to embrace life's challenges with courage and grace.

Sources:
- Vierk, Kerstin A., et al. "Prevalence of self-reported food allergy in American adults and use of food labels." Journal of Allergy and Clinical Immunology, vol. 119, no. 6, 2007, pp. 1504–1510.
- Boyce, Joshua A., et al. "Guidelines for the diagnosis and management of food allergy in the United States: Report of the NIAID-sponsored expert panel." Journal of Allergy and Clinical Immunology, vol. 126, no. 6, 2010, pp. S1–S58.
- Sicherer, Scott H., and Hugh A. Sampson. "Food allergy: Epidemiology, pathogenesis, diagnosis, and treatment." Journal of Allergy and Clinical Immunology, vol. 133, no. 2, 2014, pp. 291–307.

Chapter 30: Garlic in the Kitchen: Tips, Tricks, and Recipes

Embark on a flavorful culinary adventure as we explore the versatile world of garlic in the kitchen—unleashing its aromatic charm and tantalizing flavors in every dish. Join me as we discover practical tips, tricks, and a treasure trove of delectable recipes that celebrate the humble garlic's culinary prowess. From selecting the finest bulbs to mastering essential techniques, let's embark on a journey that will elevate your cooking to new heights of flavor and satisfaction.

Practical Tips for Working with Garlic in the Kitchen
Unlock the secrets to handling garlic like a seasoned chef with practical tips that will streamline your culinary endeavors. Learn the art of peeling garlic cloves effortlessly, mastering the mincing technique for maximum flavor extraction, and preventing garlic from burning during cooking. Discover ingenious tricks for removing garlic odor from your hands and kitchen utensils, ensuring a seamless and aromatic cooking experience every time.

How to Select, Store, and Prepare Garlic for Cooking
Navigate the garlic aisle with confidence as we demystify the selection, storage, and preparation process for this culinary staple. Learn to identify high-quality garlic bulbs based on their firmness, plumpness, and absence of sprouting. Explore optimal storage methods to preserve garlic's freshness and flavor, whether in the pantry, refrigerator, or freezer. Master essential techniques for peeling, chopping,

slicing, and crushing garlic with ease, unlocking its full potential in your culinary creations.

Creative Culinary Uses for Garlic in Various Dishes and Cuisines

Ignite your creativity in the kitchen with innovative ways to incorporate garlic into a wide array of dishes and cuisines. Explore the aromatic nuances of roasted garlic in creamy dips and spreads, savor the bold flavors of garlic-infused oils and dressings, and elevate classic recipes with a burst of garlic essence. From Italian pasta dishes and Mediterranean-inspired salads to Asian stir-fries and Latin American marinades, discover endless possibilities for enhancing your favorite recipes with the irresistible allure of garlic.

Collection of Delicious Garlic-Based Recipes for Appetizers, Entrees, and Sides

Indulge your culinary senses with a curated collection of mouthwatering recipes that showcase garlic's starring role in every course. From savory appetizers like garlic butter shrimp and bruschetta to hearty entrees such as garlic herb-roasted chicken and garlic-infused pasta dishes, delight in the robust flavors and aromas that garlic brings to the table. Complement your main courses with irresistible garlic bread, roasted garlic mashed potatoes, and garlic-infused vegetable sides, creating a symphony of flavors that will captivate your taste buds and leave you craving more.

As we embrace the culinary magic of garlic in the kitchen, let us revel in the joy of cooking, savoring each moment as we create delicious memories and share unforgettable meals with loved ones. For in the vibrant cloves of garlic, we find not only the essence of flavor and aroma but also the inspiration to unleash our creativity and passion for cooking, one delicious dish at a time.

Sources:
- Kuo, Grace, and John A. Ashton. "Garlic in traditional medicine." Food and Agriculture Organization of the United Nations, 2003.
- Block, Eric. Garlic and Other Alliums: The Lore and the Science. Royal Society of Chemistry, 2010.
- Yagi, Akira, et al. "Antioxidative defense mechanisms against reactive oxygen species in erythrocytes." BioFactors, vol. 8, no. 1-2, 1998, pp. 51–54.

Chapter 31: Growing Garlic at Home: A Beginner's Guide

Embark on a rewarding journey of garlic cultivation right in the comfort of your own home with this comprehensive beginner's guide. Join me as we explore the step-by-step process of growing garlic in home gardens or containers, from planting to harvesting. With seasonal tips, pest management strategies, and troubleshooting advice, you'll soon be enjoying the bountiful harvest of flavorful garlic straight from your own backyard.

Step-by-Step Instructions for Growing Garlic in Home Gardens or Containers

Discover the joys of growing garlic from start to finish with easy-to-follow instructions tailored for beginners. Learn how to select the best garlic bulbs for planting, prepare the soil for optimal growth, and plant garlic cloves at the ideal depth and spacing. Follow along as we nurture garlic plants through each stage of growth, from sprouting green shoots to developing robust bulbs ready for harvest.

Seasonal Planting and Harvesting Tips for Different Garlic Varieties

Unlock the secrets to successful garlic cultivation with seasonal planting and harvesting tips tailored to your region and climate. Explore the ideal planting times for different garlic varieties, whether hardneck or softneck, and discover the optimal growing conditions for each type. From autumn planting for winter harvests to spring planting for summer harvests, adapt your garlic growing schedule to maximize yields and flavor.

Common Pests and Diseases Affecting Garlic Plants and How to Manage Them
Navigate the challenges of garlic cultivation with insights into common pests and diseases that may affect your garlic plants. Identify troublesome invaders such as aphids, onion maggots, and fungal pathogens, and learn proactive strategies for prevention and control. Explore natural remedies, organic pesticides, and cultural practices to safeguard your garlic crop and ensure healthy, thriving plants throughout the growing season.

Troubleshooting Tips for Common Garlic Cultivation Problems
Empower yourself with troubleshooting tips and solutions for common garlic cultivation problems that may arise along the way. From yellowing leaves and stunted growth to garlic bulbs that fail to form or split prematurely, troubleshoot issues with soil fertility, watering practices, and environmental conditions. Harness the knowledge and expertise needed to overcome challenges and nurture your garlic crop to success.

As you embark on your garlic growing journey at home, embrace the satisfaction of nurturing plants from seed to harvest and savoring the flavorful rewards of your labor. With this beginner's guide as your companion, you'll cultivate a thriving garden full of vibrant garlic plants and enjoy an abundant harvest of fresh, aromatic bulbs to elevate your culinary creations.

99

Sources:

- Ellis, Barbara W., et al. "Garlic." University of Vermont Extension, 2003.
- Bryant, M., et al. "Garlic Production." University of Georgia Extension, 2015.
- Hannebaum, K. "Garlic Growing Guide." PennState Extension, 2018.

Chapter 32: Preserving Garlic: Techniques for Long-Term Storage

Delve into the art of preserving garlic and unlock the secrets to prolonging its shelf life while retaining its flavor and nutritional value. Join me as we explore a variety of methods—from traditional to innovative—for preserving garlic through drying, freezing, pickling, and fermenting. With expert guidance and practical tips, you'll discover how to savor the vibrant essence of garlic year-round, enhancing your culinary creations with its distinctive aroma and taste.

Overview of Methods for Preserving Garlic
Embark on a journey through the diverse landscape of garlic preservation techniques, each offering unique benefits and applications. From classic methods used for centuries to modern approaches adapted for contemporary kitchens, explore the full spectrum of options available for extending the shelf life of fresh garlic while enhancing its versatility in cooking.

How to Properly Store Fresh Garlic to Prolong Its Shelf Life
Master the art of storing fresh garlic to preserve its quality and flavor for extended periods. Learn essential tips for selecting the best garlic bulbs for storage, ensuring optimal conditions for maintaining freshness and preventing premature spoilage. Explore the ideal storage environments, whether in a cool, dry pantry, a well-ventilated cellar, or a dedicated garlic keeper, to safeguard your garlic harvest and enjoy its culinary benefits year-round.

Techniques for Drying, Freezing, Pickling, and Fermenting Garlic

Discover an array of preservation methods that capture the essence of garlic while extending its shelf life for long-term enjoyment. Explore the art of drying garlic cloves to create fragrant garlic powder or delectable garlic chips, perfect for seasoning a variety of dishes. Experiment with freezing garlic in convenient portions, preserving its flavor and aroma for use in soups, sauces, and marinades. Dive into the world of pickled garlic, infusing cloves with tangy brine and aromatic spices for a delightful addition to salads, charcuterie boards, and appetizers. And embrace the ancient tradition of fermenting garlic, transforming it into probiotic-rich garlic paste or black garlic with complex flavors and health benefits.

Tips for Maintaining Garlic's Flavor and Nutritional Value During Preservation

Unlock the secrets to preserving garlic's distinctive flavor and nutritional profile throughout the preservation process. Discover techniques for blanching garlic before freezing to retain its color and texture, optimizing the quality of frozen garlic for future use. Explore best practices for selecting vinegars, spices, and other ingredients for pickling garlic, ensuring a harmonious balance of flavors and preserving its natural goodness. And delve into the art of fermentation, harnessing beneficial bacteria to enhance garlic's digestibility and unlock its full potential as a culinary and medicinal ingredient.

As you journey through the world of garlic preservation, embrace the opportunity to savor its vibrant essence year-round, enriching your culinary repertoire with its aromatic charm and nutritional benefits. With these techniques for long-term storage at your fingertips, you'll enjoy a bountiful harvest of preserved garlic delights, elevating your cooking to new heights of flavor and satisfaction.

Sources:
- UC Master Gardeners of Napa County. "Preserving Garlic." UC Master Gardeners of Napa County, 2018.
- Vetter, J. "Garlic: Postharvest Operations." Food and Agriculture Organization of the United Nations, 2006.
- National Center for Home Food Preservation. "Garlic." University of Georgia, 2020.

Chapter 33: Garlic Supplements: Choosing Wisely for Maximum Benefits

Set off on your journey through the world of garlic supplements and unlock the secrets to choosing wisely for optimal health and wellness. Join me as we navigate the landscape of garlic supplementation, from selecting high-quality products to understanding dosage recommendations and safety considerations. With expert guidance and insights, you'll gain the knowledge needed to harness the full potential of garlic supplements and reap their maximum benefits for your well-being.

Guide to Selecting High-Quality Garlic Supplements
Navigate the maze of garlic supplements with confidence as we uncover key factors to consider when choosing the right product for your needs. Learn to identify reputable brands known for their commitment to quality, purity, and efficacy, ensuring that you invest in supplements that deliver tangible results. Explore essential criteria, such as standardized allicin content, manufacturing processes, and third-party certifications, that distinguish superior garlic supplements from inferior alternatives.

Understanding Different Forms of Garlic Supplements, such as Capsules, Powders, and Extracts
Delve into the diverse array of garlic supplement formulations available on the market, each offering unique advantages and applications. Explore the pros and cons of capsules, powders, liquid extracts, and aged garlic preparations, considering factors such as bioavailability, convenience, and shelf stability. Gain

insights into the various extraction methods used to isolate garlic's active compounds, from steam distillation to cold pressing, and their impact on supplement quality and potency.

Dosage Recommendations for Garlic Supplements Based on Intended Use
Unlock the secrets to optimizing the therapeutic benefits of garlic supplements through personalized dosage recommendations tailored to your specific health goals. Whether seeking cardiovascular support, immune enhancement, or overall wellness, discover evidence-based guidelines for determining the appropriate dosage and duration of supplementation. Explore recommended dosages for different garlic preparations, ranging from standardized allicin supplements to aged garlic extracts, based on clinical studies and expert consensus.

Safety Considerations and Potential Side Effects of Garlic Supplementation
Navigate the potential risks and side effects associated with garlic supplementation with a comprehensive overview of safety considerations. Explore common concerns such as garlic breath, gastrointestinal upset, and allergic reactions, and learn how to minimize these effects through proper dosage titration and administration. Gain insights into potential interactions between garlic supplements and medications, herbs, or dietary supplements, and consult with healthcare professionals to ensure safe and effective integration into your wellness regimen.

As you embark on your journey of garlic supplementation, empower yourself with knowledge and discernment, choosing wisely to maximize the benefits for your health and well-being. With this guide as your companion, you'll navigate the complexities of garlic supplements with confidence, unlocking their full potential to support your journey towards optimal vitality and vitality.

Sources:
- Lissiman, Elizabeth, et al. "Garlic for the common cold." Cochrane Database of Systematic Reviews, no. 11, 2014.
- Khatua, Taraknath, et al. "Garlic and cardiovascular disease: A critical review." Journal of Nutrition and Food Sciences, vol. 5, no. 6, 2015.
- Ried, Karin, et al. "Garlic Lowers Blood Pressure in Hypertensive Individuals, Regulates Serum Cholesterol, and Stimulates Immunity: An Updated Meta-analysis and Review." Journal of Nutrition, vol. 146, no. 2, 2016, pp. 389S–396S.

Chapter 34: Incorporating Garlic into Everyday Life: Practical Tips and Ideas

Enjoy making discoveries as we explore creative ways to weave the aromatic charm and health benefits of garlic into your daily life beyond the confines of the kitchen. Join me as we uncover innovative applications of garlic in self-care routines, household tasks, and holistic wellness practices, enriching your life with its multifaceted properties and versatile uses.

Creative Ways to Incorporate Garlic into Daily Routines Beyond Cooking
Unlock the full potential of garlic as a versatile ingredient that transcends culinary boundaries, infusing everyday routines with its distinctive aroma and flavor. Explore creative ways to incorporate raw or cooked garlic into breakfast, lunch, and dinner recipes, from hearty omelets and savory sandwiches to vibrant salads and flavorful stir-fries. Discover the art of garlic-infused beverages, such as refreshing garlic lemonade or invigorating garlic tea, to kick-start your day with a burst of energy and vitality.

Garlic-Infused Self-Care Products for Skin, Hair, and Oral Health
Elevate your self-care rituals with the aromatic allure of garlic, harnessing its nourishing properties for radiant skin, lustrous hair, and vibrant oral health. Explore DIY beauty recipes featuring garlic-infused oils, masks, and scrubs to cleanse, moisturize, and rejuvenate your skin naturally. Embrace the invigorating benefits of garlic-infused hair treatments, from strengthening masks and scalp massages to stimulating hair growth

and enhancing shine. And unlock the secrets of garlic-infused oral care products, such as mouthwashes and toothpaste, to promote gum health and fresh breath with every smile.

Household Uses for Garlic in Cleaning, Gardening, and Pest Control

Transform your home into a sanctuary of health and vitality with the natural cleaning and gardening prowess of garlic. Discover homemade cleaning solutions infused with garlic extracts or essential oils, effectively banishing germs, odors, and stains while minimizing environmental impact. Embrace the power of garlic in organic gardening practices, from deterring pests and enhancing soil fertility to promoting plant growth and resilience. And explore eco-friendly pest control strategies featuring garlic, such as garlic spray for repelling mosquitoes, ants, and other unwanted visitors, ensuring a harmonious balance between nature and nurture.

Innovative Ways to Enjoy the Health Benefits of Garlic Outside of the Kitchen

Expand your horizons and embrace the holistic wellness potential of garlic beyond its traditional culinary roles. Explore innovative applications of garlic in holistic health practices, such as aromatherapy and herbal medicine, harnessing its aromatic essence and therapeutic properties for relaxation, rejuvenation, and vitality. Discover the ancient art of garlic therapy, from garlic foot baths and poultices to garlic steam inhalations and aromatherapy diffusions, to promote overall well-being and harmony of body, mind, and spirit.

As you integrate the aromatic allure and health benefits of garlic into your everyday life, embrace the transformative power of this humble yet potent herb to enrich your holistic wellness journey. With practical tips and ideas to inspire your creativity and curiosity, you'll embark on a path of discovery, vitality, and abundance, guided by the timeless wisdom of garlic's multifaceted gifts.

Sources:
- Winston, David, and Steven Maimes. Adaptogens: Herbs for Strength, Stamina, and Stress Relief. Healing Arts Press, 2007.
- McGee, Harold. On Food and Cooking: The Science and Lore of the Kitchen. Scribner, 2004.
- Gohil, Kashmira J., and Jagruti A. Patel. "A review on Bacopa monniera: Current research and future prospects." International Journal of Green Pharmacy, vol. 4, no. 1, 2010, pp. 1–9.

Chapter 35: The Future of Garlic: Emerging Research and Potential Discoveries

Set sail on a journey into the cutting-edge realms of garlic research, where scientists and scholars unravel the mysteries of this ancient herb and uncover its potential for revolutionary discoveries. Join me as we explore current trends, exciting advancements, and future possibilities in garlic science and technology, illuminating pathways towards innovation, health, and sustainability in the years to come.

Overview of Current Trends and Advancements in Garlic Research
Immerse yourself in the dynamic landscape of garlic research, where a wealth of knowledge and innovation is reshaping our understanding of this humble yet remarkable herb. Explore current trends in garlic science, from molecular biology and phytochemistry to clinical research and agricultural practices, illuminating the multifaceted dimensions of garlic's biological activity and therapeutic potential. Gain insights into recent breakthroughs and key findings that drive the field forward, paving the way for transformative applications in medicine, nutrition, and beyond.

Exciting Areas of Study Exploring Novel Uses and Applications of Garlic
Journey into the frontier of garlic research, where scientists and researchers push the boundaries of innovation to unlock new uses and applications for this ancient botanical treasure. Explore exciting avenues of investigation, from exploring garlic's role in immune modulation and gut microbiome health to investigating

its potential applications in sustainable agriculture and environmental remediation. Delve into interdisciplinary collaborations and cross-cutting research initiatives that harness the synergistic power of garlic's bioactive compounds for addressing pressing global challenges and enhancing human health and well-being.

Potential Future Discoveries in Garlic Science and Technology
Peer into the crystal ball of garlic research and envision a future brimming with promise and possibility, where groundbreaking discoveries await on the horizon. Anticipate potential breakthroughs in garlic science and technology, from elucidating novel bioactive compounds and mechanisms of action to developing innovative delivery systems and cultivation techniques. Envision the integration of garlic-based therapeutics into precision medicine approaches, personalized nutrition strategies, and holistic wellness regimens, unlocking new frontiers in preventive and personalized healthcare.

Implications of Ongoing Research for the Future of Garlic-Based Medicine and Nutrition
Reflect on the transformative implications of ongoing research for the future of garlic-based medicine and nutrition, where ancient wisdom converges with modern science to shape a healthier, more sustainable world. Consider the potential impact of garlic-derived pharmaceuticals, nutraceuticals, and functional foods in preventing and managing chronic diseases, promoting longevity, and enhancing overall vitality. Explore the ethical, social, and economic dimensions of integrating garlic-based interventions into healthcare systems and dietary practices, fostering resilience, equity, and

empowerment across diverse communities and cultures.

As we gaze towards the future of garlic, let us embrace the spirit of curiosity, innovation, and collaboration that propels scientific inquiry forward, illuminating new pathways towards health, wellness, and sustainability for generations to come.

Sources:
- Lawson, Larry D., and Wallace J. Dillard. "Garlic: A Review of Its Medicinal Effects and Indicated Active Compounds." In Phytomedicines of Europe, edited by Iqbal Ramzan, pp. 177–209. Springer, 1998.
- Rahman, Khalid, et al. "Garlic 2000: A Review of the Medicinal Uses of Garlic." In HerbalGram: The Journal of the American Botanical Council, no. 49, 2000, pp. 32–51.
- Bayan, Leyla, et al. "Garlic: A Review of Potential Therapeutic Effects." Avicenna Journal of Phytomedicine, vol. 4, no. 1, 2014, pp. 1–14.

www.ingramcontent.com/pod-product-compliance
Lightning Source LLC
Chambersburg PA
CBHW070819260726
48660CB00005B/1910